NO ABSENCE OF MALICE: THE MEDICAL CULLING OF AMERICA

ALEX BURKE

CONTENTS

FOREWORD

During my research and investigation of the criminal activities going on in health care, the Obama health initiative was being hotly debated. Most people seriously doubted whether or not the bill would ever clear the House and Senate, let alone become law. Now that it has become law, the debate continues although it has changed in scope.

During the 2012 presidential elections, the Republicans claimed they wanted to repeal the law, even Mitt Romney said he wanted to do something about it, which was a very interesting position considering he was one of the main architects of health care reform and had established its predecessor in Massachusetts while he was governor.

Since the election, the first phase of Obamacare has been implemented with more changes on the way. At this critical juncture, it's time that Americans face some hard facts. One main fact has to be mentioned at the outset.

The Federal government has now become our doctor. Whether we like it or not, whether we care to admit it or not, that's exactly what has happened.

To some people, that fact may not be such a bad thing. Some people believe that whatever the government does, it has our best interests at heart. However, recent events in this country should prove quite emphatically that is not the case. If anything, we should all be put on notice that we have been lied to, and our health and futures have been compromised.

We have to realize that the government is now practicing medicine and without a license. The government will decide on our care, how we receive it or even if we "qualify" to receive that care.

By 2014, significant changes in health care and how we get that care will be well underway making the current medical landscape unrecognizable. We've heard all the promises about what the legislation contained, and we've relied on Main Stream Media to break it down so that we would understand how it would impact our lives. Certainly the administration and Congress knew that such a massive bill, over two thousand pages, wouldn't be read completely by the average American. In fact, it would be difficult to find anyone in Congress who has read the bill in its entirety.

Still, they knew our reliance on sound bites would be our main source of information. Believing those promises proposed by the administration and putting our trust in the media has more or less given Washington a free hand in dismantling American health care as we know it. In its place it has established a vehicle for the culling of Americans.

If you think that statement is over the top or over-reactive, let's look at the real facts that are contained in the legislation and you might just change your mind. The information might very well save your life.

Up until now, we had the freedom to choose our own doctors, hospitals and clinics, to accept or to reject treatments and prescriptions. While the system was not perfect, American medical care was the best in the world. Even though insurance companies have made things confusing, difficult and annoying, by and large we had access to remarkable care.

Doctors were free to order tests, to discuss with their patients the course of treatments and options. Patients were free to see the doctors of their choice. That was under the freedom umbrella, which no longer exists, in spite of what we've been told.

The new legislation has brought to the forefront, what previously has been alluded to, disguised and even denied. America is dangerously close to full blown socialism and there's no denying it. Unless Americans act swiftly and demand a change, there will be no escape.

One of the major planks in building a socialist country is through its health care. Once the freedom to choose medical care and the ability to receive that care have become arduous, the building of the socialist framework in the remaining areas of our lives will move swiftly placing the country under lockdown.

Vladimir Lenin knew this quite well and said, "Socialized Medicine is the keystone to the arch of the socialist state."

Obama knows this equally well and his health care victory is really a victory in the battle between freedom and communism. While other major inroads have been made in our country's makeover, this book will focus only on the atrocities of "health care" under the new regime.

At first blush, the health care legislation seemed to be an answer for those without insurance, those underinsured and those suffering from previous or exempted conditions that made getting insurance next to impossible.

Basically, Americans were not given a clear picture of what the legislation would really do, how it would affect our wallets, our health and our lives. That was completely intentional on the part of the administration and the media.

Major changes were intentionally put off until after the 2012 election to ensure an Obama victory. Once his second term began, all hell broke loose. Doctors now have been tasked with making new kinds of decisions, not merely about treatments and patient well-being, but now they have to decide whether or not a patient should be treated or helped to die.

That is no exaggeration. A weighted questionnaire has been developed that is supposed to help doctors determine if their patients qualify for treatment. Are they over age 60? What is their quality of life? How expensive are the treatments and prescriptions that would be used to keep those patients alive?

As discussed later in the book, the Hippocratic Oath has been rewritten to the extent that taking lives is "permissible." Nevertheless, the new guidelines for doctors have excoriated most physicians' concepts of healing. Doctors have been forcibly placed on death panels that supposedly never existed.

New doctors thinking of challenging the status quo might find it difficult to obtain licenses and established doctors might be prohibited from renewing their licenses. This is only one of many questions arising for American doctors. The prospects of the new health care have made doctors rethink their position about staying in medicine.

Many doctors are now contemplating early retirement because the practice of medicine has been altered so dramatically under the new law that patient health and well-being is challenged on nearly every level. In essence, doctors' hands are tied. Doctors who care about their patients and their treatment will find it nearly impossible to live out their ideals under the new structure. Consequently, by 2020, it is estimated that there will be a shortage of 90,000 doctors in this country.

Not only are the new regulations making it unnecessarily hard for doctors to practice medicine, but the reimbursements for doctors' services will be significantly less. In many instances, doctors will not be able to keep their doors open due to lower reimbursement rates because the doctors won't make enough money per hour to pay their staff and office overhead.

As a result, some doctors are now moving to Chile to practice medicine where they can find the freedom to treat their patients the way they should be treated. Areas of specialization will also be fewer due to major reimbursement cutbacks that apply specifically for specialty medicine. In fact, there will be no difference in reimbursement for doctors who are general practitioners or specialists.

Another large group of doctors will no longer be able to take Medicare or Medicaid patients because the government has taken $718 billion out of Medicare. Countless patients, those already dependent on government assistance will not be able to find doctors to treat them. Worse, Medicare Supplemental insurance premiums went up 22% under the new regulations. For this reason, fewer people on Medicare will get treatment, but conversely, more people on Medicaid will be treated, if they can find a physician.

Discrimination against the elderly? Most certainly that is the case. Even prescriptions for the elderly will be limited and eventually cut off.

With fewer doctors, that means longer waiting periods in obtaining treatment. In some areas of the country, the average wait to see a doctor is now four months. In one case, a woman needed a Pap smear and it took 11 months for her to get the appointment. Once you do get to see the doctor, the waiting room wait could be as long as twelve hours, while the actual time spent with the doctor will be greatly reduced.

The farcical health care solutions will force some doctors to "cherry pick" patients who are healthier and need less care in order to survive. Healthier patients mean bonus points for physicians.

To whom can the sicker patients turn?

The recent results of a survey of doctors provides good insight into the shape of medicine today and in the near future leaving no doubt that we're hitting critical mass.

If we think that our doctor can't or won't see us, we can always go see another provider. Right? That might not be as easy and you think. Of the doctors surveyed, 60% said their practices are full. They have no room to take on new patients.

Of the doctors surveyed, 70% are not happy with the new legislation. No doubt the restraints and new guidelines imposed by the government have a great influence on their answers.

A whopping 80% of doctors surveyed said they can no longer take any more Medicare patients, while an even greater percentage of doctors said they can no longer take Medicaid patients.

With regards to patient/doctor time, 60% of the doctors responded that they don't have enough time now to spend with their patients.

What's the government's answer?

The shortage of doctors will be handled by the government in ways that are designed to bring marginally trained providers into the system. The state of California has taken measures to redefine who a doctor is.

While physician's assistants and nurse practitioners can in most cases take up the slack by opening independent practices, some states are implementing the use of teachers as medical personnel who will supposedly be "trained" to diagnose mental health and behavioral disorders, a disconcerting thought. Other states are now giving optometrists and pharmacists the title of primary care providers. Are those decisions in the best interest of patients?

Doctors that decide to stick it out could find it necessary to join a hospital as an employee, a bad omen for patients. Hospitals can then dictate treatment based on government guidelines and perks, good for the hospital, but bad for the patient. A critical aspect of the doctor/patient relationship will be compromised because of the conflict of interest that would exist with the doctor and the hospital. The doctor will no longer have the ability for independent and critical assessment of the patient. This is due to the reimbursement plan for hospitals, which will receive Relative Value Units. Those units go down when doctors spend too much time with their patients or order too many "unnecessary" tests.

The government is hoping more doctors leave their practices and work for hospitals. There is better control of the patient and the doctor. Additionally, as employees, doctors' hours will be set. This is a particular problem for rural patients who might not find a doctor working after 5 PM. The end result of this unholy alliance between the hospital and the doctor will make it much harder for patients to receive adequate care while retaining their right to privacy.

To further complicate the issue, no new hospitals can be built without government approval. Even expansions to existing hospitals will not be permitted without prior government consent. Under the new law and with the idiotic restrictions placed on hospitals, it is estimated that by 2030, 30% of all existing hospitals will be gone.

Obamacare has taken on an ominous role. Bureaucrats will now define the value of a person. This paves the way for the mass extermination of the disabled, elderly and those terminally ill. Cancer patients will have rationed treatments and if they are over a certain age, the treatment plan can be changed to enable their deaths.

Patients whose answers fall within the "culling" criteria will be counseled about ending their lives and be prompted to establish a new kind of living will and doctors are required to assist their patients in making these deadly decisions.

Even healthy patients lose critical rights especially with the mandatory implementation of electronic records. Further, all American citizens will have to receive RFID chips by December 2017. The chips will contain patient history, ID information along with financial information.

Proponents say that the chips will make it easier for people to receive proper care in less time, particularly when a patient is unconscious. However, when exposed to certain EMF signals, the implanted chips can burn a person and the lithium battery can also cause serious skin irritations. Yet, that is not the worst side effect.

Fondness for the so-called convenience of the chip is overshadowed by the darker aspects that have been intentionally left out of the hype. What most people don't understand is that the chips can kill. One Saudi inventor designed an RFID chip that contains cyanide so that when the recipient gets out of line, a lethal dose will be released causing a most agonizing death.

A doctor who doesn't want to administer the quality of life questions and engage in end of life discussions with patients won't be a problem. If that patient is a burden on society all that is required is a radio signal to release the cyanide. Simple and to the point, the patient's death can be attributed to "natural" causes.

Overall health care will be rationed under the new law. The limit for an individual is $5,000. For families, the limit is $10,000. Considering the price of health care, one trip to the emergency room could easily go over the limit. Health care commissioners, mere laymen in most instances, will decide what's medically best.

What can a person do?

The government now controls private health care. Just check out page 72 of the legislation and you'll see that we lost even more rights. Health commissioners have been appointed to decide on what benefits we might receive. Further, non-medical government employees working in administrative health care positions will have access not only to our medical records, but also to our financial records, including direct access to our banking records. Check out pages 56-59 in the legislation.

As of June 2013, Obama released new regulations that will force state, federal and local agencies along with any health insurers to "swap" our personal health information and opt in to join a new health care program. Personal Health Information or PHI is supposedly protected information, but this new set of regulations indicates that is not the case.

Care to opt out of the government program? It will cost you. People who do not have government approved insurance will be taxed.

Relying on our employers to provide insurance is not a safe bet either. Companies that self-insure their workers will now find the government has the right to audit the companies' books at will. Many companies have already stated that it's cheaper to pay the government imposed penalties rather than to pay insurance premiums. Of course, they could always hire illegal aliens who will automatically get health care.

As it stands now, 7 million people will lose employer based insurance. If we think NAFTA hit American workers hard, this will hit even harder.

Americans that don't have employer based health care benefits are finding their insurance premiums are going through the roof. One individual was paying $700 per month to insure her family and that premium jumped to $2,000 per month for the same coverage.

Obama supposedly did well among college students in the 2012 election. However, if they'd known that their insurance premiums would skyrocket after the election, the outcome might have been different. In New Jersey all college students must have insurance in order to enroll.

It's clear even after just a preliminary look at the new health care that hardly anyone is left out when it comes to being targeted either in the wallet or in care. Yet, there's one group of people that is completely exempt from the new health care mandates. How do we get into such an elite group? Simple. Run for the Congress or the Senate.

If the health care act was so remarkable, why would Congress even need an exemption? The answer is obvious. It's so bad, no one would willingly want it.

Undoubtedly, high costs in health care have led to a system that is out of control, which needs an overhaul, but many doctors believe this could have been accomplished without the help of the government.

For instance, it is not uncommon to find extraordinary overbilling by hospitals who justify the practice claiming it offsets services provided to the uninsured. Hospitals have been known to charge at least six times the actual cost of pills, pacemakers, bandages etc. The price of a pacemaker is around $9,000. But some hospitals have charged insurance companies as much as $100,000 for the same pacemakers.

Pills prescribed by doctors for hospital patients get an enormous mark up. Often the actual price for one dose of a pill is about $1 to $5 dollars, but hospitals charge as much as $145 for each pill. Consequently, insurance companies balk at paying much of the bills and even if they do pay, the insurance premiums go up dramatically to help them to defray the costs.

It is criminal what some hospitals will do and the loser is always the patient.

Some doctors in Oklahoma have suggested that hospitals revamp their system. Hospital administrators and administrative employees rake in inordinately high salaries only adding to budget problems. Of course, those administrators would rather increase their salaries and maintain job security than to run an efficient hospital. The extra administrative personnel don't add to the efficiency of the hospital whatsoever.

To prove the point, a group of doctors in Oklahoma run their own surgical clinic. They keep costs way down, the business is run efficiently and patients not only get better care, but get much more personal attention. There is no reason that hospitals couldn't learn from their example. From what research has shown though, hospitals are not very inclined to change and with the new regulations, there is even less incentive.

Doctors have suggested that hospitals use transparent pricing and cut redundant or excess services that only drive up total costs to patients, but add nothing to patient care. It will be interesting to observe how hospitals will do under the new regulations.

Some hospitals are getting very competitive in their pricing when it comes to playing ball within the health exchanges that have been implemented. One such hospital that brought about some consternation was

Kaiser Permanente in California. When health care "reform" first was introduced during the Nixon administration, Kaiser Permanente was the driving force behind the whole scheme. President Nixon's good friend, Edgar Kaiser, ran Kaiser Permanente, whose main philosophy was to give less care in order to gain more profits. HMO's were born paving the way for the bureaucratic infection that would overpower health care in this country. This has been covered in detail later in this book. Suffice it to say, it is a chilling account of how Americans were sold out.

Kaiser Permanente is still up to its old tricks. A recent article in the Los Angeles Times noted that Blue Cross of California was offering individual coverage at $287 per month, while Kaiser was charging $325 for the same coverage.

We have seen in recent reports that the government is targeting certain groups within this country. Health care is no exception. American gun owners have been targeted under the new law. Larry Pratt, the executive director of Gun Owners of America, a lobbying group, stated about the legislation, "It says that all of our medical records are available to be pawed through by bureaucrats somewhere in Washington, looking for a reason to disenfranchise gun owners."

Considering recent IRS targeting of TEA Party members, pro-life groups and other conservatives, it appears the government is setting unconstitutional precedents quite readily.

It would take volumes to list all the problems with the new health care and still not cover the real reason behind it all. This book was written to expose the truth of what is driving all these changes and how it will affect each one of us.

Sadly, we are worth more dead than alive. Through exhaustive research, this book details the secret plans of a relatively small group of people who have orchestrated the deadliest plot against humanity. While many nationalities have been targeted, Americans are being targeted in a much broader and deadlier way.

Through vaccines, prescriptions and even our water and the air we breathe, we are being placed under total control of those who want to eliminate 90% of the world population. In this book, the methods will be discussed at length. Additionally, there are case studies of people that have been caught up in this scheme, but don't think that any of us is immune to such treatment.

We are all being targeted only most of us are unaware of it. A major element used in this war against us is to medicate us for normal circumstances in life. Just look at all the commercials that are aimed at treating all sorts of disorders, but did you know that the majority of those disorders are fictional? This is covered in depth in a following chapter. However, a good description of the overall goal can be found in one succinct statement from Bertrand

Russell. It gives us a macabre overview of the initial plans of the "new" health care. He said, "Diet, injections, and injunctions will continue from a very early age to produce the sort of character and the sort of beliefs that the authorities consider desirable...and any serious criticism of the powers that be will become psychologically impossible"

We will be programmed to feel, to think and to act only in the ways authorities deem tolerable. If we do not go along with the program, the authorities have a cure for that too. In order to understand the inherent nature of these plans, we have to realize that we are viewed as commodities, expendable ones at that. This book explains the sinister plot established by psychiatrists in the 1960's and covers the chilling details about how well that plot has taken hold. Did you know that the psychiatrists involved in secret meetings have developed a way to totally control our behavior?

Our children are especially at risk under the new health care. Parental rights are being stripped away with greater regularity, a necessary part of the overall plan. We are losing even the most basic human rights and yet the majority of us are silent. Why? Main Stream Media have a significant role in only reporting the party line and leaving out the most crucial details. Consequently, people are tuning out and becoming less engaged in the day-to-day news, which only augments the control placed on us.

By looking at real patients, unfiltered facts and allowing ourselves to be educated, we can see a much clearer picture of just what is at stake. The people mentioned in this book tell a story much more eloquently than any news program. Their stories could easily become our stories at the mere twisting of an ankle, a seemingly little fall or any minor injury.

We can go on believing in what the media has been paid to say or we can listen to those who know first-hand about health care and where it's going in the US. We can turn our backs only so long before we are confronted with our own medical crisis. Either through age, through injury or illness, we're all on the same road.

The people in this book can tell us about our present and future condition. If, however, we decide to close our minds, our ears and our hearts to the new reality and not heed the warnings sounded so clearly, we have no one to blame but ourselves. We can continue to doubt the degree to which this nation has fallen or we can arm ourselves with the truth and make the necessary changes to guarantee our future.

CHAPTER ONE
FIRST: DO HARM

Something is horribly wrong with the health care system in our country. In Ohio, for instance, record numbers of doctors are turning on their patients in direct violation of the Hippocratic Oath. Often this betrayal leads their patients into a physical and emotional ordeal filled with anguish and depression. In many cases, it leads to their deaths. What might motivate doctors to do this?

To comprehend what is going on in the Ohio health care industry and in health care systems at large, it is important to understand a network that fosters unethical behavior and even rewards it. Doctors are crossing the line without a second glance, breaking the law and breaking the trust their patients place in them.

Except in a few instances, law enforcement shrouds itself from the corruption that is taking place. Supposedly, internal review boards investigated claims of abuse, but found no malfeasance. Was that the case?

Evidence uncovered during an initial investigation by Doctor Robert K. Nichols, an Ohio chiropractor, contradicted those assertions and proved collusion and duplicity involving several state agencies, private corporations and elected officials on the local, state and federal levels. The investigation revealed undue influence by major corporations over state agencies and managed health care providers in order to maximize the highest gains possible, estimated in the billions of dollars per year.

Dr. Nichols discovered a complex web of deceit and fraud that resulted in the deliberate abuse of patients and in some cases, their needless deaths.

He uncovered the major role some doctors had in this scheme and the lengths to which they would go. Therefore, it is critical to explore the deadly game these doctors play with their patients and their systematic bastardization of medicine.

In order to grasp the extent of this corruption, it is also important to look at specific patients and the trauma to which they were exposed at the hands of those men and women sworn to help them.

The focus of this book is to reveal the things that have happened to people within the Workers' Compensation program in Ohio. However, the problems and abuses are not inherent to Ohio alone, but are also present in other states. Many of the corporations that handle managed care for injured workers in Ohio have offices in several states. Anywhere managed care organizations operate can be a dangerous place to fall ill.

Doctor Nichols was in the perfect position to uncover the systematic abuses on the part of the Bureau of Workers Compensation or the BWC and the managed care corporations or MCOs. Some of his patients suffered greatly because of the machinations of a system rife with criminal activity.

Nichols promised his patients and himself that he would fight for them against a system that let them down. Those patients, desperate to find relief, could only think about getting rid of their pain and trying to get back to work. As a chiropractor, Nichols could do a great deal for his patients with specific treatments, but he could not prescribe medication for them. He had to refer his patients to pain management doctors within the BWC system.

Pain medication was all too easily approved, but surgery to fix the injuries was not. As an injured worker's tolerance to a particular medication built up, the pain returned and often injuries were aggravated. Some employers, the BWC or managed care providers pressured patients to return to work even though their conditions were not improved, causing even more dependence on powerful pain medications. Corrupt doctors intentionally misdiagnosed serious injuries as strains or sprains when in fact the patients had herniated discs in the neck and spine. When diagnosing supposedly simple strains and sprains, no MRIs are ordered. Therefore, it is impossible to tell if the injured worker is more seriously hurt. The investigation uncovered that the doctors did this deliberately and at the behest of the BWC.

Some doctors choose this shortcut because payouts for simple diagnoses are expedited, whereas complicated diagnoses delay payments to the doctor. As further investigations revealed, this is a necessary part of the overall scheme to defraud employers at the expense of the injured workers and taxpayers. A more detailed look will be covered in a later chapter.

Injured workers are left to languish in limbo. A debilitating cycle can develop that could lead to severe depression and anxiety, and if not treated effectively, could result in the body turning on itself. When that happens, it leads eventually to organ failure.

These realities motivated Nichols to find out the cause for the BWC's negligence and what he discovered convinced him that he had to turn on his own for the sake of countless patients suspended in a system without hope or relief.

He launched a campaign to help his patients and others to find the assistance they needed so badly and ultimately he hoped to find them justice.

Their fight became his fight, their pain virtually became his, nearly consuming him. Dr. Nichols found out quickly that he was battling powerful adversaries who sought his destruction anyway possible.

Through bureaucratic pressure, they tried to shut his practice down by delaying and appealing his compensation for treatments. He nearly lost his practice, but managed to keep it afloat, yet not before it cost him tremendously.

Dr. Nichols is compassionate and cares about other people's suffering. He went to Chiropractic school to become a doctor patients would trust and one who saw the person, their suffering and not his bottom line. Nichols is an anomaly in Ohio health care, one that his enemies would like to see stopped.

After writing a book about health care reform, Dr. Nichols' life started to disintegrate. His colleagues were not pleased that he had written such a scathing evaluation of his peers and the health care system. Nichols turned an intense light on those whose practices could not hold up under the scrutiny. Nothing happened to those doctors. Instead, the focus was shifted to Dr. Nichols.

Nichols came home one evening to find his computer had been hacked and the message on the screen was clear. He had to stop what he was doing or suffer the consequences.

After thinking seriously about the warning, he decided to continue the fight. The stakes were high. If Nichols went forward, revealing what was happening, doctors throughout Ohio, the BWC and managed care providers stood to lose millions of dollars.

They launched counter-measures against him in hopes their crimes would not be revealed and their cash cow would not be slaughtered.

Nichols did not focus on or think too long about the power of his enemies and the lengths they would go to stop him. In his mind, he saw what was right and wrong. He saw the faces of his patients and the other injured workers who were suffering terrible torments.

It drove him to the brink of obsession. Dr. Nichols spent endless hours compiling information, making phone calls and trying to go through channels to help his patients.

Still, the system railed against him and stepped up the game, placing him under investigation, and questioning his billing practices.

Although no irregularities were found, the sheer stress and pressure seemed intolerable not only for Nichols, but also for his wife and family.

Bonnie Nichols worked with her husband in his office and was well acquainted with the questionable tactics of the BWC and the managed care providers. Nichols knew the toll of the job took on her.

After one of Nichols' patients died unnecessarily due to bureaucratic red tape, she decided it was enough and found another job at a local hospital.

The BWC further tightened the screws. When the compensation payments to Nichols were held indefinitely, they lost their home, and the family of four had to move into a cramped two-bedroom apartment.

They barely had enough to eat, but still Nichols pushed the system for answers. He would not relent and his patients loved him and supported him. In fact, when he could no longer afford to feed his family, Nichols' patients, poor themselves, donated what money they could to help him.

His patients knew he was fighting the good fight right beside them. They understood his struggles and they formed a bond that proved impenetrable.

Nichols sought help and advice from lawyers and former prosecutors familiar with the tactics that the BWC used against him. They warned him about the dangers of what he was doing and they told him that the powerful people behind the Bureau and MCOs would come after him using whatever means they had.

One former prosecutor that had gone up against the same people met with Nichols secretly to give him a specific warning. This attorney related some things that happened to him when the people involved decided to make his life a living hell.

Consequently, the attorney went into hiding. He gave up his cell phone, credit cards, and bank accounts, anything that would aid this group in hunting him down. He told Nichols to be careful and suggested that he forget about pursuing his investigation because, "These people will kill you."

After a warning like that, most people would have reevaluated their position and probably would have given up. Dr. Nichols would not give up. He would not let his patients down.

Somehow, deep inside he found what he needed to go on and to help the patients who depended upon him. He had to do something beyond what he had tried before, even though it was incredibly dangerous. Even though the retaliation could cost him his life, Nichols risked everything and decided to do something extraordinary.

CHAPTER TWO
THERAPEUTIC NIHILISM

Finding himself in the position of fighting for his life, and the lives of his patients, Nichols had to come to terms with a nightmare. He had to find a way of confronting his enemies directly. Nichols had to find something that would help him to fight a battle that was foreign to him.

Nichols did not know if he had the courage or the bravado to continue, but he did know he had to do something quickly.

After he was followed to and from work, after his patients were followed to and from his clinic, Nichols was backed into a corner. From there he could give up, ignore his patients' plight and the fraud that was taking place or he could fight.

When some of his patients told him what happened during their periodic Independent Medical Exams or IMEs, he knew he had to take action. Doctors would barely examine the injured workers; some did not examine them at all and reached a diagnosis that the people were fit to return to work, when clearly that was not that case.

Nichols checked on the reports the doctors submitted to the BWC and found them contradictory to what his patients had experienced, but to change the status quo, he had to find a way to prove the doctors' deception and scheme. At this stage, Nichols had no idea just how much the corruption had metastasized within the system.

To find out just how pervasive the problems were, he decided to get the doctors on videotape and he recorded phone conversations with the BWC and MCOs that would prove without a doubt the presence of corruption.

Nichols decided to get a video camera and give it to his patients that had Independent Medical Exams or IMEs scheduled so they could videotape their own exams without the doctor's knowledge.

Faced with the problem of legality, Nichols researched the Ohio Code to determine whether the videotaping was legal. He thought he found the precedent he needed. Just to make sure he was correct, he asked for legal opinions from lawyers and an Ohio State Senator, John A. Boccieri, who is now a United States congressional representative.

Senator Boccieri had the Ohio Legislative Service Commission do the research. Under the law, there are particular rights associated with ownership of the property and the issues of the power to exclude.

According to the code, "The power to exclude has traditionally been considered one of the most treasured strands in an owner's bundle of property rights."[1] The law states that an owner of either residential or commercial property has every right to exclude persons from that property.

The finding stated, "Property does not, however, lose its private character merely because the public is generally invited to use it for designated purposes."[2] Therefore, any company or office has the authority to deny anyone access to the property. In the Commission's letter to Senator Boccieri, it stated, "Any right of access to the property that a customer or client does have must be 'Balanced against the constitutionality secured rights of the property owner.'"[3]

The letter further stated, "Nothing in the Revised Code prohibits customers or clients from making video recordings on business property, but barring other factors, an owner or lessee of property both may exclude persons from their property and prohibit persons from making a video recording while on their property."[4]

Nichols got his green light to videotape the exams. He also checked into the legality of taping phone conversations and found two precedents, one in the US Code[5] and the other in the Ohio Revised Code[6] that allowed for one person in the conversation to tape the call without the other's consent.

It also occurred to him that he could prove why some injured workers, including his patients, died waiting for treatment. He looked up the statistics going back to 2000 and through 2006. The numbers shocked him.

---

[1] Bresknick v. Beulah Park Limited Partnership Inc. (1993), 67 Ohio St.3d 302, 303; Loretto v. Teleprompter Manhattan CATV Corp (1982) 458 U.S. 419, 435
[2] Cincinnati v. Thompson (1994) 96 Ohio App. 3d 7, 17; Lloyd v. Tanner (1972) 407 U.S. 551, 569
[3] Thompson, 96 Ohio App. 3d at 17
[4] January 3, 2008 Letter to Senator Boccieri from Ohio Legislative Service Commission
[5] 18 U.S.C. §2511
[6] Ohio Rev Code Ann. §2933(b)(4)

The graph below shows the number of Injury Related deaths as opposed to Non-Injury Related deaths.[7] The Non-Injury deaths occurred while injured workers were being treated or in most cases waiting for treatment to be approved. Some non-injury deaths were associated with accidental drug overdose from inordinate amounts of medication, suicide, and organ failure brought on by depression that stemmed from the injury. Often ancillary illnesses that were byproducts of their injuries such as heart attacks brought on by stress contributed to the cause of death.

An alarming disparity exists between the two categories. For example, while there were only 171 Injury Related deaths that occurred in 2006, 8,108 Non-Injury Related deaths occurred.

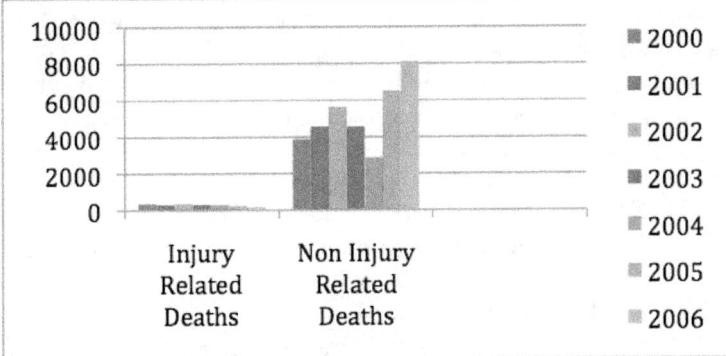

Nichols thought he knew why these people died while under the BWC's and/or the MCOs watch. He hoped he was wrong, but his instinct said otherwise. Still, he needed to prove it. After he found out that some of his patients were scheduled for their IMEs, Nichols asked them if they would agree to take the video camera with them to record the exam. When some of his patients agreed to videotape their mandatory exams, he knew eventually that he could compile a compelling case that would rock the system and the state of Ohio. Nichols hoped it would make a difference before any more people died unnecessarily.

He knew his investigation would show why honest and caring doctors had their hands tied by the BWC and were prevented from treating their patients and operating on them in a timely fashion.

One surgeon, after seeing a patient with a horrible knee injury, was distraught because the BWC would not pay for the badly needed surgery. He told the patient that his case would be the last Workers' Compensation case he would take. The doctor added that he got into medicine to help people and the BWC prevented him from doing the right thing.

---

[7] Data provided by the MCO ADR Department at the Bureau of Worker's Compensation

Dr. Bruce Siegel, a Cincinnati doctor and pain management specialist, was in agreement about the BWC abuses. He worked for the BWC until the 1990s and really understood the questionable practices within the organization. Siegel said, "They do not give a darn whatsoever what happens to the worker. They will pay their doctors to say whatever is necessary to postpone payment, to deny payment, or to put it off as long as possible. I've seen some ridiculous responses to them."[8]

Dr. Siegel, considered a pariah by the BWC, went on to condemn MCOs saying that they "make money for the company and nobody else at the expense of the patients' health."[9]

While these doctors' opinions were revealing, Nichols knew they were not enough to prove the corruption going on within the agencies. However, Nichols felt that if he exposed the inner workings of the system, change would have to come. The doctors who really cared about their patients would be able to treat them, and the corrupt doctors would finally pay for their malfeasance and would be drummed out of medicine.

As the patients went through their exams and returned with the videotapes, Nichols was convinced that he was on to something. He was appalled to see the gross negligence on the part of the doctors and their pseudo exams.

Some exams lasted only three minutes without the doctor even examining the patient's injuries. Doctors asked the patients cursory questions, but did very little hands on examinations.

Nichols followed up by getting copies of the reports that the doctors filed and they confirmed the fraud. Doctors billed the BWC for much more extensive exams. In many cases, the doctors fabricated information.

Whereas the doctors benefited greatly from these exams, the patients suffered further distress. Their needs were not addressed and the superficial exams in most instances did not result in the patients getting their surgeries and necessary treatments approved. In fact, the BWC carries the dubious honor of denying 97% of all claims. The playing field was never level and the injured workers rarely stood a chance of getting real help.

The pain and the systematic abuse overwhelmed beleaguered patients. Some sought the help of an attorney, and as Dr. Nichols found out, another door opened up that led to further corruption.

Nichols had patients that went to lawyers for help with their Workers' Compensation cases trying to get the assistance in navigating the system. However, some of the lawyers did little or nothing for their clients. When it came to representing these patients at hearings, the lawyers barely showed up.

---

[8] The Blade-Blade Investigation: BWC Scandal Riles Claimants; Injured Workers See Millions Lost As They Fight for Help
[9] The Blade-Blade Investigation: ibid

If they did arrive on time for the hearing, they would not fight for their clients, preferring to accept, without question or argument, the decision of the hearing officer. Even if that meant the decision went against their clients unjustly, the lawyers did nothing.

Thwarted by lack of funds and the inability to travel to other cities to find representation, many of Dr. Nichol's patients went to lawyers in their own area. This often seemed pointless. All too often, the patients never spoke to the lawyer, but rather to a representative.

Phone calls to the law offices were not returned, escalating the frustration and helplessness the patients felt. Without competent legal representation, injured workers fell prey to the BWC and suffered for it financially. To Nichols, it appeared that some lawyers were part of the BWC's racket. Some of his patients felt that the lawyers were getting kickbacks from the BWC.

Injured workers were forced to file for bankruptcy due directly to the BWC's willful negligence and malfeasance. By not permitting the proper therapy or surgery, injuries did not heal, and the bureaucratic process extended to the point of absurdity. Therefore, workers could not return to their jobs in a reasonable timeframe.

The longer an injured worker stays within the system, the monetary rewards increase exponentially for the agencies, but not for the injured workers. The agencies have a stake in drawing out the whole process, bilking the injured workers' employers by ordering IMEs and going through the hearing process that could take years for which the employer is financially responsible. Then the premium rates increase for Workers' Compensation insurance for employers, which can drive many businesses to go under because the cost of staying in business is too great. With today's economy, that is especially true. Ohio has been hit particularly hard in the crisis, with the exception of the BWC and MCOs that continue to flourish.

The BWC was doing so well that millions of dollars were thrown into some questionable investments that opened another door to even more fraud. An investigation revealed a crooked trail leading to some well-placed politicians, who will be discussed later. This confirmed to Nichols that he was on the right road.

Nevertheless, he could not jump safely into the fray without careful planning, and so he continued to gather videos, taped phone conversations and documents building a foundation his enemies could not destroy.

The results are compelling accounts of the people caught in a veritable trap with little hope of escape, caught within a system broken beyond repair. This is their story, but in it heartbeat, it could also be ours.

CHAPTER THREE
FOR THE GOOD OF MY PATIENTS

In discussing the abuses of injured workers caught up in the BWC and MCO whirlwind, it is imperative to look at how the MCOs make their money and to understand why inhumane decisions are made at the expense of the injured worker's welfare and sometimes at the cost of his life.

The MCOs drive injured workers literally into a dubious process that takes them on a path of inefficient care, and quite often, the care is three times as costly. The substandard care compounds the difficulties of the workers in not only their ability or more often in their inability to heal, but also by adding psychological sequelae, or the conditions that follow an injury, complicating the situation. Consequently, the injured workers are forced to go through the appeals processes and reviews. That drives more money into the MCOs.

The final goal is to have the workers declared disabled so that the MCOs can place them in their Voc-Rehab programs, where the MCOs get the big money from a surplus fund. Rarely do the injured workers benefit from the process. Normally, the workers get the run around and not the training they need, but the MCOs get their money regardless.

With this belabored process, benefits are lost frequently and severe depression sets in. Obviously serious issues arise when workers who live paycheck to paycheck end up without any means of support. They have to resort to legal action to get their issues addressed.

In 2005, according to the BWC, 258,308 issues were taken to hearings.[10] Of those issues, 90% of the cases heard at the first level of hearings were appealed.

On the surface that might seem like a good thing, but if we look at what an injured worker has to go through just to get help, and the time and expense involved, it can be highly detrimental.

For any particular issue, it takes forty-five days to have a hearing. In addition, there is a fourteen-day appeal process with another seven-day appeal period to have the MCO decision appealed -- and that is merely to get a hearing for the issue in the first place.

It gets worse. There is another forty-five day period for a second hearing. That is well over ninety days with financial responsibilities looming over the injured workers; their homes often fall into foreclosure. This normally happens well before any decision is made about receiving or reinstating benefits. Even if the Physician of Record or POR says the injured worker needs those benefits or treatments, it does not seem to matter.

Therefore, the injured workers lose any means of support; with it they lose their homes, their vehicles and all too often, their dignity. While the MCOs rake in obscene amounts of money, injured workers find themselves at square one, still hurting badly from their injuries, still seeking help that may never come.

For a closer look into this unethical environment, we can focus on specific injured workers and their journey through the jungle of corruption. One of the best examples is Bill Durst, pictured below.

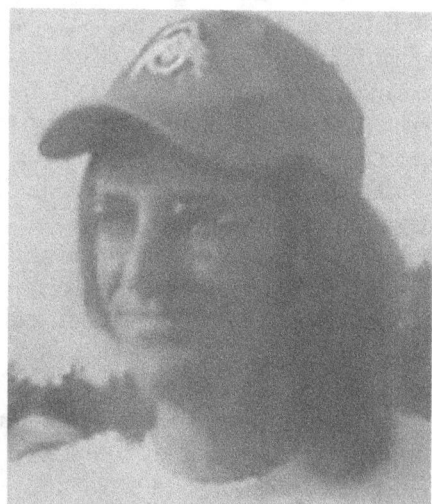

Bill Durst 2006

---

[10] Industrial Commission Motions and Appeals Filed in 2005 according to volume per docket.

Mr. Durst, husband, father and grandfather, worked for a tire company. One day at work, a friend and co-worker was caught in between furnaces when a fire broke out and the emergency release lever at the exit failed to operate. Mr. Durst and his co-workers finally extricated the man from the fire, but it was too late. The man burned to death. The company was sued and subsequently shut down.

Not content to draw unemployment, Mr. Durst found a job working for Temporary Personnel Services located in Minerva, Ohio. He was 42 years old, healthy and in the prime of his life. On August 14, 2002, he was sent to a job in Pennsylvania to unload tires from a semi-trailer. While unloading it, he lost his footing and fell onto the blacktop several feet below. He hit his head and back. Although he was in severe pain, an ambulance was not called. When Mr. Durst finally got home that day he was in agony.

His wife, Debbie, took him to Alliance Community Hospital in Alliance, Ohio. A nurse put him in a wheelchair immediately, fearing he had a serious back injury. She told him not to move. Then Mr. Durst was taken into an examining room where a doctor gave him a curious exam.

He was moved to a gurney and placed directly on his back. The emergency room doctor took Mr. Durst's legs, bent his knees and brought them up towards his chest. Mr. Durst screamed in intense pain and offered some choice words to the doctor. The doctor chastised him for his "bad bedside manners." The doctor told Mr. Durst he was bruised. The doctor did not order any X-rays or CT scans. No bone scans and no MRIs were ordered. He was sent home without treatment.

With the doctor's diagnosis, Mr. Durst thought he could return to work, but he was still in terrible pain.

Perhaps concerned about liability with Mr. Durst's injuries, his employer offered him an office position in one of their other offices that did not require any lifting or too much physical exertion, "pushing paperclips," as Mrs. Durst recalled. The office was an hour drive from his home. Needing the money, he decided to try it.

The trip to the satellite office was grueling and he told his employer he could not stand the pain of the drive back and forth. In fact, Mr. Durst could not tolerate sitting or standing for any length of time. The employer then recommended that he drive 15 minutes, pull over and rest 15 minutes and then drive another 15 minutes until he got to the office.

After four days, Mr. Durst had to quit because he could not handle it. The employer, however, achieved his goal of appearing magnanimous to Mr. Durst. It is unfortunately common practice to put the injured worker in a stressful situation. Some employers hope that they will quit, and in some cases do all they can to get injured workers to quit, which would end their financial responsibility to the employee. Certainly, it was not only stressful, but also extremely painful for Mr. Durst.

Seeing her husband in horrific pain, Debbie Durst was not satisfied with the diagnosis. She took her husband to see Dr. Nichols because she thought he could help.

Nichols later related his examination. He said, "I could tell from the amount of pain he was in and the total lack of movement (Range of Motion) he had with his back, neck and shoulder. I performed orthopedic tests that most everyone has learned in either chiropractic or medical school and arrived at the conclusion that he couldn't have any manipulation until he had X-rays on his low back along with an MRI and follow-up bone scan. I needed the scan to determine whether or not the fracture was recent or old."

After the results came back, Nichols saw the fracture in the lumbar region was recent. It was diagnosed as a pars interarticularis fracture. The bone scan also found a fracture of Mr. Durst's iliac crest or pelvic bone and vertebra. According to Nichols, that was caused by the fall and hitting the blacktop.

Following his assessment of Mr. Durst's condition and going over the results of the tests that were performed, Nichols treated him with passive care using inferential current and ice to decrease the swelling, inflammation and pain.

It was obvious to Nichols that Mr. Durst needed to see a neurosurgeon, but he had to go through BWC channels. Mr. Durst was able to see Dr. Mark A. Weiner in Canton, Ohio on January 15, 2003. At that time, Dr. Weiner agreed that Mr. Durst had a fracture of "part of the vertebrae called the pars interarticularis" and recommended that he have cortisone epidural injections, which were widely used treatments for that condition.[11]

Mr. Durst got approval finally to have the cortisone injections and he was scheduled to have three sessions that were intended to alleviate the pain. During the first session, Mr. Durst nearly passed out from the pain of the injections into his lower back. He mustered the courage to go to the next treatment, but in the middle of it, the doctor stopped because he said it would harm Mr. Durst even more and he could not finish the mandated sessions.

Dr. Weiner saw Mr. Durst again and said that he needed surgery to place rods and a plate in his back. The procedure, an L5 laminectomy and fusion, allows two bones to fuse together to keep the bones and joints from moving. He told Mr. Durst that he was aware of the obstacles in getting that done through the BWC. Dr. Weiner also told Mr. Durst to do everything he was asked to do by the BWC so that surgery would not be put off.

The protocol with this surgery entails six weeks of post-surgery recovery to allow the bones to fuse and then rehabilitation can start. Therapy normally

---

[11] March 12, 2003 letter from Dr. Mark A. Weiner, MD

continues for six to eight weeks and by the end of six months, the patient is recovered generally.

However, CareWorks, the managed care organization handling the Durst case for the BWC, did not go along with the doctor's assessment. The first request for surgery was denied, but Mr. Durst's pain level increased. He was placed on heavy-duty narcotics just to make life tolerable. Mr. Durst continued to see Dr. Nichols for treatment to help him handle the pain, while he waited for the BWC to give permission for the surgery.

Mr. Durst's battle for surgery continued. He tried to get specific therapies to help him, which were often denied. Yet, he easily got more and more pain medication. Mr. Durst had to jump through hoops that no injured worker should ever have to attempt. Still, in order to reach the surgery carrot dangled in front of him by CareWorks, he had to go through the mandatory steps.

It was Mr. Durst's great misfortune to have his health care directed by CareWorks, the largest managed care firm in Ohio. The founder of CareWorks, William Pfeiffer, was a former BWC administrator and a top aide to the former Democratic House Speaker Vern Riffe. Not surprising then that CareWorks received more than $347 million dollars from the BWC from 1997 through 2006.

During that time, the firm managed to sign 33% of the 5,821 public employers as clients. However, being the largest managed care firm did not make it the best. In fact, CareWorks was rated as the worst MCO in Ohio, not only in total claims driven into the litigation process, which numbered 19,238 for the period from 2000 to 2004, but also as the worst provider for total cost to employers for processing appeals.[12]

Within the period of 2000-2004, CareWorks charged employers nearly $4 million for the litigation process. The figures below show the Top Five Worst Ranked MCOs for the timeframe.

Managed Care Organizations	Total Claims Litigated
CareWorks	19238
CompManagement Solutions	16590
Sheakley	10937
Gates-McDonald Health Plus	8601
CorVel	3983

---

[12] MCO and BWC Disputes Received January 1, 2000 through December 31, 2004 for MDs and DCs.

Managed Care Organization	Cost of Appeals to Employers
CareWorks	$3,847,600
CompManagement Solutions	$3,318,000
Sheakley	$2,187,400
Gates-McDonald Health Plus	$1,720,200
CorVel	$796,600

These numbers are considered relatively modest and are quite likely doctored on the part of the MCO's, but they do give an idea of the situation detrimental not only to the injured worker's employer, but also to the injured worker.

Once in the hands of CareWorks, Mr. Durst found himself in a vicious and repetitive cycle of doctor visits, hearings and the royal runaround that led to his loss of benefits. On one such cycle, his benefits were pulled arbitrarily and his house went into foreclosure. He and his wife had to put the house up for sale hoping not to lose all of their investment.

Just as the final days ticked down on the foreclosure, his attorney was able to secure his benefits and their house was saved. Still, Mr. Durst's condition deteriorated.

In agony, he was given even stronger pain medication for his injuries, but CareWorks would not budge on the surgery. They told Mr. Durst that he could not have surgery until all treatment avenues were exhausted.

Dr. Nichols tried to help him anyway he could, but the BWC and CareWorks refused. This was also during the period that Nichols was under constant scrutiny from the BWC. Due to his complaints about the system, the BWC made every move very difficult for Nichols and for his patients.

Three times Nichols put in the request to get Mr. Durst the treatments he needed. Each time CareWorks denied the very treatments they had stipulated were required prior to surgery. Three times Mr. Durst got his hopes up and three times, he was denied.

This torture continued without relief, without surgery and without hope of returning to a normal life. During this period, Mr. Durst, an already thin man, lost even more weight. Once a man with a healthy appetite, he eventually ate far less than his 3-year-old grandson. He grew severely depressed and no longer cared about taking care of his appearance.

Mrs. Durst said that CareWorks "stripped him of his manhood" and beat him down. The pain, a constant and cruel companion, became worse. Playing ball with his son, Billy, was no longer possible. He lost interest in almost everything. Yet, the family kept fighting and hoping that CareWorks would approve the badly needed surgery.

In the midst of this fight, Mrs. Durst had a fight of her own. She was diagnosed with colon cancer and needed surgery. Mr. Durst tried to be there for her at the hospital and did what he could, but things did not go smoothly. Mrs. Durst developed a massive infection that nearly killed her.

She finally recovered and had to return to work, albeit too soon, because the family desperately needed the income. At this point, Mr. Durst was fighting yet another round with CareWorks and trying to cope with the pain and frustration.

CareWorks still did not approve therapy or surgery, but continued to approve high-end painkillers.

In order to cope with the pain, doctors told Mr. Durst to take acetaminophen or Tylenol in between his regular pain medications in hopes he would be more comfortable.

After a long period of trying to find the right pain medication, Mr. Durst wound up so heavily medicated that he could hardly walk and often his wife would have to pick him up off the floor after he had fallen, further aggravating his back. His legs would become numb, and the pain even more unbearable, but still no surgery was authorized.

CareWorks documents dated 09/24/04 that were obtained through this investigation stated that the company would not approve Mr. Durst's surgery due to a lack of medical information. Was there really a lack of information?

A letter from Dr. Mark A. Weiner, dated 09/08/04 contradicted that assertion. Dr. Weiner stated specifically in his letter that Mr. Durst needed an L5 Gill laminectomy and fusion. He further stated that Mr. Durst had undergone several modalities or treatments without any "lasting benefit." Consequently, surgery was the remaining option for him.

Was Mr. Durst a malingerer in the eyes of CareWorks and that is why they refused the surgery? Often the BWC and MCOs tend to view injured workers as fakers or malingerers trying to milk the system. While there have been people that have filed bogus claims, the majority of cases are legitimate.

In view of what his doctors stated in their records and in light of the kinds of prescriptions they prescribed, it was obvious they did not agree with the BWC. Even to untrained eyes, the medical evidence alone was more than sufficient proof of Mr. Durst's injuries.

Doctors in charge of pain management for Mr. Durst finally prescribed a skin patch called Lidoderm Lidocaine, 5% every twelve hours. The prescription called for two patches to be worn, but Mr. Durst did not always use them. Taking several medications for pain and the subsequent depression that followed, he did not want to take any more medication unless it was necessary. There are serious side effects associated with the drug such as lightheadedness, tremors, nervousness, respiratory distress or arrest and "cardiovascular manifestations may include bradycardia, hypotension and cardiovascular collapse leading to arrest."[13]

As the issue of surgery went unresolved, and as the constant pain started to beat down Mr. Durst, he saw a psychologist, William. D. Diorio, Ph.D., LISW in October 2003. He continued to see him through 2006.

After thirty-five sessions with Mr. Durst, Dr. Diorio gave his opinion about his condition. Dr. Diorio stated that Mr. Durst suffered from "unremitting moderate symptoms of the Major Depressive Disorder, as causally and inextricably associated with multiple physical injuries, have combined to result in a degree of functional impairment that renders Mr. Durst permanently and totally disabled and unable to engage in any gainful employment, including skilled sedentary work."[14]

Dr. Diorio's opinion agreed with Dr. Nichols' opinion of November 29, 2005, which stated that Mr. Durst "is unable to perform sustained and remunerative employment and found to be permanently and totally disabled."

By the lack of CareWorks response and the failure to set a date for the Mr. Durst's surgery, it is evident that the company did not care about his pain or his severe depression causally related to his injuries. His mental health started to deteriorate because he could not escape the pain.

Dr. Diorio's assessment[15] of Mr. Durst's mental state at this time consisted of the following:

1.   He is depressed most of the day, every day.
2.   He suffers from insomnia: difficulty falling asleep and staying asleep.
3.   There is a marked reduction in his level of psychomotor activity, as self-reported and validated over time through observation in sessions of psychotherapy.
4.   He struggles with and against chronic fatigue, with low energy levels every day and significant reduction in activities of daily living.
5.   There is a marked and persistent reduction in appetite; he is thin and physically weak.
6.   There is marked loss of sexual interest, desire, with impairment in sexual response.
7.   He has pervasive feelings of worthlessness and guilt because he is unable to work, earn an income and adequately provide financial support for his family.

[13] http://www.drugs.com/pro/lidoderm.html
[14] Letter from William D. Diorio, Ph.D LISW to Nikitas Skoufatos, Attorney-at-Law, Durst Attorney
[15] William D. Diorio, PhD sent a letter dated May 14, 2006 to Nikitas Skoufatos, Attorney-at-Law, Durst Attorney

8.   He often feels "trapped" and "overwhelmed," unable to concentrate, reason clearly, with his level of intelligence, cognitive functioning, and occupational position, prior to becoming injured and clinically depressed.

From the lack of CareWorks approval for treatments and surgery, Mr. Durst went from a healthy and vital man to one that could barely make it from moment to moment. His family also had a difficult time not only in the day-to-day challenges of making ends meet, but also in watching someone they love deteriorate.

Dr. Diorio said that Mr. Durst was always, "a faithful and dedicated worker, with a strong work ethic and commitment to 'perfection' in all aspects of his life." Therefore, Mr. Durst must have been overwhelmed in the position in which he found himself. Dr. Diorio's description of Mr. Durst and his willingness and need to work should have confirmed to CareWorks that he was not trying to defraud the system, but needed immediate help. Still, CareWorks would not approve the surgery.

In his July 18, 2006 letter to CareWorks, Dr. Diorio requested more sessions for Mr. Durst because his depression was worsening. Diorio stated that it was cheaper in the end to approve the treatments than to keep up with the "costs of expensive psychotropic medication or psychiatric hospitalization." Diorio was worried about his inability to "maintain Mr. Durst's resilience and mental stability over time, in the face of his chronic pain and physical disabilities."[16]

After Mr. Durst saw a psychiatrist, Nicholas A. Atanasoff, DO, it was reconfirmed that Mr. Durst was now totally disabled because of his major depression.

Doctors were concerned because of Mr. Durst's deepening depression because they knew the effects on the body and the risks for significant cardiac problems. He was on a downward spiral encouraged by CareWorks medieval approach to patient care.

A psychiatrist, Dr. Anil Choudary Nalluri, MD, administered the Zung's Depression Scale to Mr. Durst, which revealed that he was suffering from severe to extreme depression. When Dr. Nalluri asked Mr. Durst if he could have three wishes, what would they be, Mr. Durst answered, "Just one: go back to 8/14/02 (the date he was injured) and stay home all day."[17]

On September 1, 2006, Mr. Durst had a tense and difficult day. His wife came home from work that evening and left shortly to pick up some dinner. When she returned, Mr. Durst told her he was not hungry. He said he was going to use the pain patches and then go to bed. At 7:30 PM, she went out to

---

[16] Letter dated July 18, 2006 from Dr. Diorio to CareWorks
[17] Report from Dr. Nalluri to Nikitas Skoufatos dated August 23, 2006

rent a movie and when she got back, Mr. Durst was still in the bedroom. She watched the movie and went to bed about 11 PM. When she got into bed, she noticed her husband was lying partially on her side of it. Mrs. Durst tried to move him, but he did not respond.

She turned on the light and looked at her husband. He was dead. Mrs. Durst became hysterical and her son, Billy, ran into the room. She tried to keep him from going over to his father, but he pulled away and saw him. Billy grew distraught.

The coroner was called and Mr. Durst's body was taken directly to the funeral home. Mrs. Durst could not afford an autopsy and waited for the coroner to hear about the cause of death. The coroner of Columbiana County, William Graham, Jr., MD, ordered a forensic toxicology blood and urine panel for Mr. Durst and subsequent to the findings, he listed the primary cause of death as myocardial infarction. The secondary cause of death was acetaminophen intoxication caused by a buildup of the drug over time.

Here was a man whose heart and blood pressure were normal until he was placed on medication necessary to treat his pain and depression, necessary because CareWorks would not approve spinal surgery that doctors felt was critical to his recovery. Records indicate that Mr. Durst had no known heart problems. However, with depression, especially as severe as Mr. Durst's, the risks of heart attack, coronary disease and sudden death increase dramatically. The serious side effects of the medication Mr. Durst was taking could cause blood clots, bradycardia and other complications, and created a deadly cocktail. This tragedy would not have transpired, if Mr. Durst had been treated properly.

Unfortunately, you do not have to be in the Workers' Compensation program today in order to experience malfeasance and inhumane treatment. Managed Care organizations are involved in treatment for people who are privately insured and their modus operandi is the same. Therefore, anyone is at risk of being treated like Mr. Durst and dying not only because of the callousness of the system, but also because of its greed.

As for the Dursts, they continue to fight and to hope to put their lives together again. They are currently involved in a wrongful death suit against CareWorks and the BWC. Mrs. Durst tried to get funeral and death benefits from the BWC, which immediately put the BWC on the defensive.

The Industrial Commission, which hears the cases concerning injured workers, found Mr. Durst had permanent total disability allowed from September 29, 2005 through the date of his death. The Industrial Commission relied on reports from Drs. Diorio, Atanasoff and Nalluri, reports that CareWorks and the BWC would not support.

When it came to the death benefits petition filed by Mrs. Durst, the bureau ordered yet another file review by a BWC doctor, Dr. Thomas G. Welch, MD.

Initially, he reported on October 22, 2008 that "it is known that patients with depression and this was an allowed condition, have a greater incidence of heart attack and even sudden death." Dr. Welch summed up his report stating that Mr. Durst's death was caused by depression and the medications he was on citing, "it is certainly a likely scenario."

The BWC was not about to swallow Dr. Welch's opinion and decided to change the doctor's mind about the possible cause of death. In an email to Dr. Welch, from a BWC nurse, Ann H., she stated, "[g]iven the specific lack of any medical records from the hospitalization which resulted on the IW's [injured worker's] death, it would seem that there is little support for any allegation," concerning the wrongful death of Mr. Durst.

Unbelievably, Dr. Welch changed his opinion at Ann's request and filed an addendum report that was dated October 27, 2008. In the report, Dr. Welch stated, that it was impossible to link Mr. Durst's death to the medications he was taking because of a lack of emergency room records. He failed to mention Mr. Durst's depression, which he had done in an earlier report.

There were no hospital records because Mr. Durst was not in the hospital at the time of his death. His body was taken directly to the funeral home.

Nevertheless, the Dursts had a medical opinion to support the wrongful death suit. It came from noted physician, Dr. Pollyea from Ohio State University. Dr. Pollyea stated in his report dated, March 4, 2009, that Mr. Durst did have significant depression that caused or greatly accelerated his heart disease leading to a myocardial infarction. He used the medical reports available to him and based his decision on medical literature that supported the link between severe depression and cardiac disease and death.[18]

Yet, the evidence was not enough for the Dursts to prevail and a District Hearing Officer who filed a report dated March 9, 2009 denied the claim.

The Dursts wasted no time in filing an appeal with the help of their attorney, Jonathan Goodman. The Dursts requested that Dr. Welch review the file once more to prove that a proper opinion was provided by the BWC.

The BWC was not happy with this decision and wanted to have the file reviewed again, but this time it bypassed Dr. Welch. The ball was tossed to Dr. Alan E. Kravitz, MD, who issued a report on March 13, 2009 recommending that the BWC deny the claim on the basis that Mr. Durst sustained only "soft tissue" injuries. This opinion was issued in spite of compelling and overwhelming evidence that Mr. Durst had suffered a fracture of the iliac crest and pars articularis. Somehow, Dr. Kravitz overlooked or failed even to look at the MRIs and countless doctor reports stating that Mr. Durst was seriously injured. Incredible as his opinion was, he went even further to suggest that Mr. Durst's depression was "brief… transient and resolved."

Perhaps this is what Dr. Siegel meant when he said the BWC pays their doctors to deny claims at any cost. Unfortunately, Dr. Kravitz went on to more

---

[18] Dr. Pollyea's report to Jonathan Goodman, Esq. Durst Attorney dated March 4, 2009

extraordinary assertions when he said that there was no cause of death on the death certificate, when that was patently false. As if the hole was not deep enough already, Dr. Kravitz concluded that Mr. Durst's depression and cardiovascular disease were not related and stated that in Mr. Durst's death, there was "not a shred of evidence of cardiac death."

Ann H. was not content to let it go at that. On March 16, 2009, she sent a fax to Dr. Kravitz, which this investigation obtained. She stated, "The lack of medical documents as the IW was found at home and also when no obvious cause of death is visible then cardiac is usually indicated – and since no autopsy to confirm, we will never be 100% certain…But also please address the depression angle – something indicating that since cardiac is not proven then presence of depression is irrelevant maybe?"

Dr. Kravitz dutifully complied and filed a report dated March 16, 2009 that depression does not normally cause cardiac death and that Mr. Durst had no evidence of heart disease or myocardial infarction. He did not mention Dr. Pollyea's report or the toxicology report done by the coroner.

Due to the gross omissions and irregularities with Dr. Kravitz's reports, Jonathan Goodman, the Durst's attorney asked that Dr. Kravitz be deposed. In that deposition, Kravitz backtracked and stated that he was unaware of any medical studies done that proved the connection between depression and cardiovascular disease, stating in the deposition that he had only read "little slices" and never read whole articles on the subject.

Yet that did not stop Dr. Kravitz from attacking Dr. Pollyea's opinion, stating, "The problem is that in the real world that [linkage between depression and cardiovascular disease] doesn't seem to exist." Eventually, the Durst's prevailed.

This case, however, proves that the BWC will stop at nothing to get opinions favorable to the agency and that its managed care providers do not care whether their decisions kill innocent people. Their bottom line is all they see.

Nagging questions persist for Mrs. Durst about why CareWorks kept denying the surgery.

For four years, Mr. Durst did everything he could to get the surgery he needed and deserved. For four years, he lived in unbearable pain. For four years, CareWorks put off his surgery, overriding qualified medical opinions that stated clearly the absolute need for the surgery. For four years, he waited for CareWorks to respond in a timely manner regarding treatment and for four years, CareWorks willingly put him through anguish.

Within ten days after Mr. Durst died, CareWorks sent out their quickest response to date. A letter to Mrs. Durst simply stated that CareWorks' responsibility toward Mr. Durst has ceased upon his death. It was over for CareWorks, but not the Durst family, still struggling to make ends meet.

When asked about how CareWorks treated her husband, Mrs. Durst said, "Honestly, I think they knew Bill needed surgery. They knew he'd be laid up and draw money." She added that CareWorks seemed to want to "Discourage people so they quit. If somebody is faking, they give up. Honestly, in pain you can't give up."

Surely, Mr. Durst's medical records and the physicians' statements on file proved he had a bona fide injury that needed surgery. Unfortunately, Mr. Durst was killed by a system whose actions were clearly inhumane and criminal. Dr. Nichols said this is an unequivocal "crime against humanity." Left in CareWorks wake is a family with little support; a family left to wonder what life might have been like, if CareWorks had agreed to the surgery. After three years since Mr. Durst's death and met with problems around the house, his wife still says to herself, "I'll call Bill and ask him what to do," then remembers he is gone. He will not be there for them.

Instead, a son will never play ball with his father; a little girl will never know her grandfather and a wife will never stop wondering why.

None of us should stop wondering or asking why managed care organizations get away with their crimes. The problem, however, lies in whether or not we are prepared for the answer.

While people might not be prepared completely, it is time to lift the veil of secrecy and reveal the perpetrators.

CHAPTER FOUR
TOO CHICKEN TO DO IT

Mr. Durst's tragic, preventable death underscores the need to shut down the Bureau of Workers Compensation and its pimps, the managed care organizations and put an end to the crimes of the prostitute doctors. Complaints filed with the BWC and the Industrial Commission which oversees the bureau, are unanswered or ignored. No investigations are launched, therefore the multitude of sins continues. Admittedly, the behemoth bureau and bureaucratic red tape have made policing its activities difficult, but not impossible.

In order to ensure that the bureau and managed care organizations are operating within and not above the law, someone with authority has to have the courage to initiate a thorough and unbiased investigation. If that cannot be done within the internal affairs of the offending agencies, then it must be addressed outside of the system, but that seems unlikely under the existing conditions in the Ohio State government. Perhaps due to the political and financial gains at stake, people in authority over the BWC seem reticent about any investigations.

The responsibility lies squarely with those higher up on the food chain to put an end to the corruption. The attorney general and governor have a definite responsibility to investigate the serious charges Dr. Nichols has leveled at the BWC and MCOs.

The governor at the time, Ted Strickland, received a copy of Dr. Nichols' book, *Broken Arrow*. In it, Dr. Nichols discusses in depth the crimes that occur within the bureau and MCO framework. It is unclear whether the governor actually read the book. According to his aide, Charles Preston, the governor was aware of the book and supposedly passed it on to a think tank of ten or fifteen people that address issues concerning the BWC and those pertinent to the governor.

In a recent call to Mr. Preston, he told the author that his position is merely to help constituents that are "badly in need of help like obtaining food stamps and other things." When he was asked about whether or not he would help injured workers obtain treatment from the BWC and managed care organizations before they died, he stammered around the subject. Reminding him that the governor's constituents include injured workers and that thousands of them die every year or commit suicide, he said that a "new director was appointed to the BWC who had great business experience and really had a tight hand in running the bureau and is doing a fine job." Mr. Preston was informed that that was not the case -- that right now injured workers are contemplating suicide because of the failures of the system. The author was then directed to contact the press secretary, whose direct responsibility includes applicable spin, but no one-on-one constituent assistance.

For the record, the governor's office never contacted Dr. Nichols about his book nor made any overtures to the BWC. Was Governor Strickland worried about his war chest, as were his predecessors?

Whatever the supposed reasons the governor had for not investigating the state workers who were and are derelict in their duty, criminal in their behavior and who have no regard for human life, those reasons do not exclude Strickland's lack of concern regarding the abundant corruption taking place within one of his agencies. Mr. Preston told Dr. Nichols in a conversation about the book, "There's a lot of information in there." As an aide to the governor, he should have passed that information along to his boss, which obligated the state's chief executive to act or to risk being complicit in the criminal activity.

There was more than enough evidence detailed in *Broken Arrow* for any right-minded individual to have concerns. We reminded Mr. Preston of that fact and he said, "Lots of wild claims are made. We didn't expect so many from Dr. Nichols right after taking office. Dr. Nichols called here many, many times." The reasons Dr. Nichols called Mr. Preston must have escaped him. It could also be that the governor's ear and those of his staff open only to financial supporters such as those within managed care and the bureau.

When pressed further about helping desperate injured workers, Mr. Preston backpedaled in rapid-fire staccato ramblings and suddenly gushed, "This is not my bailiwick." Since Mr. Preston speaks for the governor that is a sorry indictment for Ted Strickland.

Mr. Durst's case and thousands like his shout for someone of integrity to do something. Unfortunately, countless cases of abuse happen daily that smack of duplicity, fraud, and dereliction of duty that set precedents for the BWC's handling of injured workers. These crimes are not just isolated incidents, but rather well established methods of abuse that guarantee the BWC and MCOs, and politicians an extraordinary amount of money.

Doctors and caseworkers attack injured workers, their credibility and their character while they sell their quackery to the highest bidder.

The case of Perry Marteney, Jr., further proves that there are those within the BWC and the MCOs that have a lack of regard for the sanctity of life and a pervasive attitude that the law and the injured worker be damned. In this case, the abuse has lasted nearly thirty years.

On August 12, 1980, Perry Marteney Jr., an intelligent, industrious 23-year-old man, was working on a roof. He fell and landed on angle iron, hyper-extending his back over the iron. His lower back absorbed the impact. From that moment on, his life changed dramatically and he discovered the dark side of the Bureau of Workers' Compensation.

Like Mr. Durst, he suffered for four years before the BWC approved his surgery. Unlike Mr. Durst, Mr. Marteney lived to have the surgery performed. However, the surgery brought about new problems that had to be addressed, and the situation was complicated by the BWC and Gates-McDonald who handled Mr. Marteney's managed care.

Gates-McDonald, you will recall, ranked fourth in the worst MCOs both in cases sent to litigation and in costs to employers. In the case of Mr. Marteney, perhaps Gates-McDonald should also rank in the top five worst MCOs in its treatment of injured workers.

Mr. Marteney's indoctrination into the BWC's tangled web started with the usual diagnosis of sprain/strain of the lower back. He was later diagnosed as having L5 Symptomatic Spondyloisthesis with instability. According to Mr. Marteney's surgeon, Dr. David W. Smith, DO, of Massillon, Ohio, it was found that the postural neural arch was "exceptionally loose and there was sizable hypertrophy of the fibrocartilaginous mass as the pars intra-articularis bilaterally." [19]

Dr. Smith performed a Spinal Fusion L5-S1, Bilateral Lateral utilizing an iliac graft from the posterior ileum. All loose fragments and the pars inter-articularis were removed. A mass of fibrocartilage was also removed at S1.

Mr. Marteney had hopes that the surgery would alleviate his pain, but subsequent to the surgery performed on October 8, 1984, he found that he had even more severe pain at the incision site that lasted for six long years. Another extremely critical fact was that the surgeon performed the wrong surgery.

The struggle for treatment and medication to combat the pain went the familiar managed care route of some approvals and many more denials for help, while Mr. Marteney fought to keep going and to keep his marriage together. It was difficult for his wife and two children to watch him go through unthinkable

---

[19] Dr. Smith's surgical report dated 10-8-84.

pain and the understandably irritable behavior from having to manage intense pain on a daily basis.

The case notes showed that Dr. Smith finally agreed to do another surgical procedure in 1990 called a Surgical Exploration Proximal to the original Laminectomy incision. It was suspected that Mr. Marteney had a Stitch Granuloma. A granuloma consists of immune cells clustered around particular substances that the body deems as foreign. In this case, Dr. Smith discovered a stitch or suture that was not absorbed by the body.

After the exploratory surgery, Mr. Marteney had 79 stainless steel staples in his low back and an 8-inch scar from his rectum up his back, adding to his original and significant distress.

Dr. Nichols described this pain saying, "Now to understand what Mr. Marteney endured for nearly six years, imagine a pin stuck in your low back and every time something, like your belt or shirt or some other garment comes into contact with it, you experience severe agonizing pain. You can't sleep because if the blanket that keeps you warm touches it or you happen to roll over onto it, you experience pain that awakens you during all hours of the night. For six years Mr. Marteney lived with constant pain."[20]

This second surgery made his pain all the worse. A third surgery was performed, but the records of it were completely expunged. The only record that the surgery had transpired was from a pathology report done during the surgery. The procedure brought no improvement either in his pain level or in his ability to function.

Records show that Dr. Smith was also a BWC independent medical examiner. In that capacity, Smith denied innumerable claims of injured workers and had numerous malpractice cases. He left Ohio quite unexpectedly, leaving Mr. Marteney in anguish.

Mr. Marteney's first marriage collapsed and his finances disintegrated. He lost his home, his car and practically everything he owned.

He received a letter from Gates-McDonald in 1992 stating that they would no longer pay for doctor visits, treatments, prescriptions or hospitalizations. This action by Gates-McDonald was standard operating procedure.

Understandably, this put an enormous psychological strain on Mr. Marteney and his second wife, Gloria. With the unrelenting, severe pain and lacking any help from the BWC, he found himself in a desperate situation. The lack of financial assistance for his treatments and medications hit the Marteney's savings account. With nowhere else to turn, Mr. Marteney could not take it anymore.

At wit's end, he attempted suicide and spent time in a mental hospital. Upon release, he tried to put his life back together, but the burgeoning pain

---

[20] Letter dated 10/12/06 from Dr. Nichols to Attorney Jonathan H. Goodman, Columbus, Ohio

made the battle difficult. Trying to get his benefits reinstated, he sought legal counsel from Webster M. Lonas, Jr. in Canton, Ohio, but that proved pointless. During several hearings, Mr. Lonas did nothing to dispute the hearing officer's position and raised no objections and as a result, Mr. Marteney lost those vital hearings. According to Mr. Marteney, Lonas was completely apathetic. The one victory he achieved came when Lonas never showed up for the hearing.

When the question of vocational rehabilitation came up, Mr. Marteney applied for it three times, and three times, he was denied. The retraining would have helped him keep active and help with the scar tissue buildup, but the bureau said he was not a likely candidate.

His records were reviewed by IME doctors that never saw him and had no idea what he looked like. They all stated that he had reached maximum medical improvement, yet this man needed to take nearly 12,000 pills per year just to survive.

One such independent medical examiner was Dr. Deborah McFarland; the clinical director of Naturally Right Chiropractic Inc. Dr. McFarland denied Mr. Marteney's claims, never having seen him, never knowing that because of the pain he suffered, he had suicidal thoughts daily. Dr. McFarland is the perfect IME doctor for the BWC because her denial rate is 97%.

Dr. Nichols went to Dr. McFarland's office to ask her about her denial rate. He carried with him hundreds of denied claims of injured workers similar to Mr. Marteney's. His camera operator went with him to record the conversation. The receptionist saw the camera and immediately went ballistic. The camera operator left the building, and when Dr. Nichols could not get in to see Dr. McFarland, he left.

Dr. Nichols asked Mr. Marteney what he thought about Dr. McFarland during a videotaped conversation, he said, "If she treats her patients like she does BWC injured workers, she can't have many patients left."

That might very well be the case. Dr. Nichols suspected there was something else going on in Dr. McFarland's office. He called her office posing as a prospective patient. The taped phone conversation was extraordinary because the secretary made a bet with Dr. Nichols that he would like Dr. McFarland's treatment and if not she would give him something to make it worth his while. One thing led to another.

Receptionist: "We'll strike up a deal. Come in here for a month and if you don't like it call back and ask for Cynthia and you and I will strike up a deal."

Dr. Nichols: "You mean if I don't like it, I can get my money back or whaddaya mean."

Receptionist: "I can't refund your money, but I can offer you something else. I'm sure of that."

Dr. Nichols: "What's that?"

Receptionist: "Well, let's bargain about that. What would you like?"

Dr. Nichols: (Uncomfortable. Laughs) "I don't know."

Receptionist: "Don't get too expressive. I gotta family at home yet. Think about it. Make it a challenge. Try it. If you don't like it, we'll do something for you."

Dr. Nichols: "I prefer pizza."

Receptionist: "I don't work weekends."

While not all IME doctors' offices are run like this, it does give an excellent example of what injured workers like Perry Marteney have to deal with when going through their independent medical exams. The lack of ethics and morality is overwhelming. If nothing else, in Dr. McFarland's case, it appeared that the stench of desperation was in the air.

From 1992 until 2006, Mr. Marteney spent $20,000 on his medical bills and prescriptions, borrowing to make payments and taking out a second mortgage on his home. The responsibility was squarely on the BWC to pay the costs that related to his original injury in 1980. Yet the bureau seemed to think everything was fine with Mr. Marteney in spite of what his physicians indicated.

His pain ratcheted up considerably and in 2006, his former mother-in-law told him to go see Dr. Nichols. He resisted at first and then finally acquiesced. After he saw Dr. Nichols and had several treatments, his pain became more bearable. Dr. Nichols helped him with the bureau to reopen Mr. Marteney's file and get them to pay for the treatments. Over time, Mr. Marteney's range of motion increased and he was able to do a few things around the home and even sleep at night. [21]

Then, the bureau did not approve any more treatments. Dr. McFarland's denial of the claim put an end to them. That was a terrible blow to Mr. Marteney. He had suicidal thoughts almost every day and did not have the pain medications he needed.

Dr. Nichols grew more frustrated with the system and tried to help him with claims, but the pressure of it all was wearing Mr. Marteney down.

In her file review, Dr. McFarland stated that Mr. Marteney should be healed, even though he had eleven allowed conditions on his claim, even though he could not work, even though the pain was so severe that he could not shut off suicidal thoughts.

Dr. Kenneth A. Jenkins said in his file review dated June 27, 2008, "This injured worker should have been healed within 25 office visits within the initial weeks following the date of injury, which as 8/12/80."[22] Dr. Nichols responded to this statement, "It seems Dr. Jenkins has found a cure for scar tissue." It would also seem that the three botched surgeries never happened.

Another medical report, this time from Dr. Charles McMarrow dated 06/14/08 said, "Chiropractic treatment records present for review are

---

[21] Dr. Nichols' case notes during 2006-2007

[22] Dr. Jenkins' 06/27/08 letter to GatesMcDonald Health Plus, Inc. Columbus, Ohio

somewhat limited in their scope and they fail objectively to support the requested services."[23]

Dr. Nichols stated, "That is absolutely untrue. My treatment is aimed at the allowed condition of post laminectomy syndrome… they are medically necessary, medically reasonable and directly and proximately related to the industrial injury of 08/12/80."

Mr. Marteney must have felt like a squashed ping pong ball bounced from one reviewer to another whose sole purpose was to deny the claims anyway possible. They failed to realize the consequences of their actions. He said, "Doctors abuse injured workers without seeing them. Nothing happens to them. Do they stop to think how many injured workers commit suicide?"

One morning, Dr. Nichols was driving to work. It was a beautiful day, the kind that makes a person glad to be alive. As Dr. Nichols drove through the Ohio countryside, he found that the scenery "Soothed my heart and mind before I walk into the office."

It was not a soothing day for Perry Marteney. To him, the day was dark and horrifically painful. Dr. Nichols recalled what happened. "I get about a quarter of the way into my tranquility and then my cell phone rings. It's Perry Marteney and he's desperately searching for a reason not to blow his brains out. I know it's bad because he's calling me in the morning and I know that his wife is working at the gas station in the mornings. He wants to do it… end the pain, the constant headaches and low back pain, and the constant pain in his groin, thighs, legs, calves and feet. The never-ending pain must stop… is what he is telling me.

"I know he's already made up his mind. I interviewed him and Gloria told me her biggest fear was that she would come home one day and find Perry dead from suicide. It was like an instant flashback to that interview. I couldn't believe it. Bill Durst said the same thing about not being able to bear the pain any longer. That was the last time I saw him alive. They cut these guys off treatment that was helping them cope with their pain.

"I told Perry not to do it. He knew that I knew he had it planned out once Gloria left. I told him not to leave Gloria or his kids, Crystal or Apryl with that memory of him. I told him that he is dealing with pure evil [Managed Care, the Bureau, and IC's Hearing Officers]. 'Don't do it, Perry,' I said, as I was approaching a dead spot in cell reception.

"My blood pressure began to rise. I told Perry to hang on and I would make them pay for the morphine pump to help stop the pain. I put myself in his shoes and doubted that I would have acted any different. But I needed him to live and told him how much his family loves him and to not leave them with the guilt not being able to help him. I told him that I filed a Criminal Complaint on the Hearing Officer that relied on the 2 bogus file reviews performed by

---

[23] Dr. Charles McMarrow medical report on Perry Marteney, Jr. dated 06/14/08

those docs and told him that I also filed Ethics Complaints on the 2 docs that did the reports and that as soon as I get to my office, I am making a phone call to the Industrial Commission's Tom Connors."

The Hearing Officer to whom Dr. Nichols referred was Clement Rogers, a trained lawyer working for the Industrial Commission. Mr. Rogers did several things within the course of Mr. Marteney's hearing for benefits that were illegal according to Dr. Nichols.

In Dr. Nichols September 9, 2008 affidavit to the Industrial Commission, he mentioned the medical reports and statements sent in by Drs. Jenkins and McMarrow were false misrepresentation of the facts "that any conscionable Hearing Officer would have challenged.

"District Hearing Officer Clement H. Rogers, in his official capacity, knowingly and intelligently under the color of law, under Ohio Revised Code 2921.12 Section (B) willfully relied upon not one (1), but two (2) alleged falsified reports/falsified medical records."

Dr. Nichols stated that Rogers had direct access to Perry Marteney's claim file evidence via on-line services right in the Hearing room. He further charged that Rogers failed "to take reasonable measures to responsibly review my office notes, which objectively and clinically demonstrated improvement in respect to this Ohio injured worker's allowed conditions of the claim ranging from improved Orthopaedic ranges of motion both active and passively, improvement in all Orthopaedic tests utilized to assess the injured worker's progress and improvement in the injured worker's capacity to function on a day-to-day basis."

Those results are upheld in the Supreme Court decision previously covered. Additionally, Nichols mentioned in the complaint that Rogers failed to consider the testimony of Perry Marteney in its entirety.

In that testimony, Mr. Marteney stated that if it were not for Dr. Nichols' treatments, he would be dead. He had every intention of killing himself to be free from pain. Dr. Nichols did give Mr. Marteney relief from some of the pain making his life more bearable.

Dr. Nichols added in his complaint, "There is no higher testament to the medical necessity of treatment provided to any patient than the reward of sustaining said patient's capacity to sustain life for which without said treatment/measures that the patient would have committed suicide."

Was Rogers truly fulfilling his responsibilities or was he guilty of Intentional Tort, which consists of malice, willfulness and outrageous misconduct towards Mr. Marteney?

The Hearing Officer must investigate in such manner as to ascertain the substantial rights of the parties and to carry out justly the spirit of such sections.[24]

Relying on reports furnished by Drs. Jenkins and McMarrow, Rogers made his decision. Was it the right one?

Let us look at the statements made by those doctors. Dr. Jenkins claimed "This injured worker should have been healed within 25 office visits within the initial weeks following the date of injury, which was 08/12/80."

Jenkins failed to mention the surgeries that were approved and paid for by the BWC. The record shows that Mr. Marteney's first surgery was on October 8, 1984. From the date of injury until that surgery there were some 217 weeks, and obviously he could not have been healed in the initial weeks following his injuries. Neither was he considered healed when his second surgery took place in 1990. Mr. Marteney in no way could be considered healed, if he had been, there would have been no need for the surgeries and the BWC would not have paid for them.[25]

Both Jenkins and Rogers must have had blindfolds on when it came to reading Mr. Marteney's file. In Jenkins case, he offered falsified information, either wittingly or because he never read the file. Whatever the reason, he brought more pain and suffering on Mr. Marteney and in doing so, violated the Ohio Revised Code. Further, Jenkins was paid for "false or misleading statements with the purpose of securing goods or services under the Workers' Compensation Act.[26]

Dr. McMarrow's file review was just as scant and full of holes. He stated that Dr. Nichols failed in his office notes to objectively support his request for Mr. Marteney to do Therapeutic Exercises. Dr. Nichols' file notes were thorough and well-documented, proving Mr. Marteney's progress and need for the treatments and as Mr. Marteney stated, he would be dead without them.

Had Clement Rogers read Dr. Nichols notes, he would have seen clearly that Dr. McMarrow was unjustified in his opinion and had no grounds to deny the claim. Dr. McMarrow violated several sections of the Code of Ethics, as

---

[24] Under 4123.10 Ohio Revised Code: The industrial commission shall not be bound by the usual common law or statutory rules of evidence or by any technical or formal rules of procedure, other than as provided in sections 4123.01 to 4123.94, inclusive, of the Revised Code, but may make an investigation in such manner as in its judgment is best calculated to ascertain the substantial rights of the parties and to carry out justly the spirit of such sections.

[25] Ohio Revised Code 2913.48 - (2) Make or present or cause to be made or presented a false or misleading statement with the purpose to secure payment for goods or services rendered under Chapter 4121., 4123., 4127., or 4131. of the Revised Code or to secure workers' compensation benefits; (B) Whoever violates this section is guilty of workers' compensation fraud.

[26] Ibid.

did Dr. Jenkins. Dr. Nichols made the State Ohio Chiropractic Board aware of these violations, but no reprimand or action was taken.

In his Ethics Complaint to the Industrial Commission, Dr. Nichols brought up crucial evidence that was completely overlooked by Clement Rogers proving that his negligence sent Mr. Marteney over the edge. Due to Rogers' alleged reliance upon falsified information, and his refusal to consider all of the evidence, he violated the Ohio Revised Code and could be found guilty of a third degree felony.[27]

The Industrial Commission took no action. When Dr. Nichols called the IC, he spoke with Barb Beazy, an assistant to Tom Connors. He told her that Mr. Marteney nearly killed himself and asked that Clement Rogers' actions be investigated. Ms. Beazy's reaction to Mr. Marteney's situation was cold, callous and inhumane. In fact, when Dr. Nichols pressed for something to be done with Clement Rogers, she chuckled.

Mr. Marteney did not carry through with his intentions, exercising tremendous courage and trust in Dr. Nichols. However, the BWC allegedly seems to be goading Mr. Marteney to carry through with killing himself.

While reading his file on the BWC Blue Dolphin site, Mr. Marteney found an entry in his file that made him reel. In the entry dated 05/18/09, when referring to a request for treatment from Ray Brunner, LISW, Mr. Marteney's therapist treating him for post-traumatic stress disorder, the entry explains Mr. Marteney is not doing well, his moods are fluctuating. Then it states, "Takes strong effort just to get out of bed. He has thoughts of wanting to die, but 'too chicken to do it.'"[28]

In an interview with the author, Mr. Marteney said he never said those words and was not too chicken because the first time he tried suicide, he nearly succeeded, and was hospitalized after the attempt. He said that comment sent him over the edge and he was advised by his doctor not to research his file because the ensuing stress and emotional upheaval was too much for him. In a compelling letter dated 06/18/2009 Mr. Marteney wrote to the BWC, he stated "When I was getting chiro treatments 3 times a week it was the best I had felt in years. Dr. McMarrow and Dr. Jenkins reviewed my claim file and basically

---

[27] (A) No person, knowing that an official proceeding or investigation is in progress, or is about to be or likely to be instituted, shall do any of the following:
(1) Alter, destroy, conceal, or remove any record, document, or thing, with purpose to impair its value or availability as evidence in such proceeding or investigation;
(2) Make, present, or use any record, document, or thing, knowing it to be false and with purpose to mislead a public official who is or may be engaged in such proceeding or investigation, or with purpose to corrupt the outcome of any such proceeding or investigation.
(B) Whoever violates this section is guilty of tampering with evidence, a felony of the third degree.
[28] Ohio BWC claim notes on Perry W. Marteney, Jr. 05/18/2009

said I was healed. A hearing officer agreed with their reports. My treatment was cut off. Dr. Nichols filed ethics complaints on both of these Drs. and [the] hearing officer not anything was done to any of these people. They were not reprimanded in any way. Dr. Nichols said that when he called in about these complaints he was laughed at. When he called the State Chiro Board, he was told by their executive director that chiros who perform claim reviews and IME are exempt from any ethics. This lack of accountability forced me to seek other treatments; the only other treatment that was recommended by my pain mgt. doctor was injections in my back. I feel I was forced into taking these injections by the bureaucracy of a system that should be helping me instead of trying to kill me. Because of the injections I have severe headaches since my 2nd epidural and these headaches are almost every day. I don't know how long I can hold on."

The BWC opted for invasive and more expensive treatment that ended up with Mr. Marteney acquiring a new disorder called arachnoiditis; this is where the outer layer of the spinal cord becomes inflamed and scars causing chronic pain and often triggers severe headaches. The condition, which was foisted upon Mr. Marteney, is not covered by the BWC. Sadly, he showed considerable improvement under Dr. Nichols care, but it appears that Mr. Marteney might be right -- that the bureau might be trying to kill him.

If we take into account Mr. Durst's case and thousands like his, is Mr. Marteney wrong? He sees where this is headed and it typifies a dangerous trend in American healthcare, especially under the control of managed care organizations like Gates-McDonald.

There is a propensity for the BWC and managed care organizations to treat injured workers and the poor with contempt, as though their existence is an offense to society. When we asked Maria Smith, the Chief Spokesperson for the BWC to investigate the claims made by Dr. Nichols and Mr. Marteney, she replied, "There is no substantive data to support Dr. Nichols' claims. The Ohio Bureau of Workers' Compensation (BWC) is committed to quality care for injured workers. We recognize prompt, effective medical care leads to a quicker recovery, timely return-to-work and improved quality of life. Each year, BWC manages claims of more than 1.4 million people. Daily, our staff exercises concerted efforts with our provider partners to provide workers with the right care at the right time with the right outcome in mind. BWC is committed to our goal of effectively meeting the changing challenges of injured workers' medical needs; as well as addressing the issues of those who are unsatisfied with decisions related to their treatment."

That statement is a disservice to the thousands of injured workers who have died waiting for treatment, or who have killed themselves to escape the pain and the pain caused to their families.

Ms. Smith was asked to review the videotaped evidence and listen to phone conversations that would prove the criminal activity within the bureau, but she failed to respond.

Governor Strickland's office was appraised of the BWC statement and asked what they planned to do to help injured workers like Perry Marteney to keep from killing themselves. Allison Kolodziej, a press spokesperson said, "We defer to the BWC that workers are treated and get what they need."

Perhaps the governor solidified more campaign contributions by keeping a hands-off approach to the fraud within one of his state agencies.

When looking at the serious plans of those who want to reform healthcare, there is indeed a movement towards implementing the practice of eugenics thereby ridding the world of useless eaters, like the injured, the poor and the sick.

However, the overwhelming abuse of the injured worker in Ohio has left the state teetering on decimation. Over 250,000 workers are hurt every year in Ohio. If they were treated like Mr. Marteney, the work force would diminish considerably. Ohio has already seen thousands of workers leaving the state because of the lack of healthcare, jobs and any hope of a future.

Governor Strickland could boast about what he is doing to change this, but the record and the facts speak for themselves. Ohio is the poster child for the annihilation of the middle class, the working class and without drastic measures and reforms; the once great state will succumb. The cause of death and the responsibility will lie directly with those within the BWC, managed care organizations and the politicians that have raped, pillaged and broken the backs of citizens they were supposed to serve.

CHAPTER FIVE
UNBRIDLED DISCRETION

It has been difficult for Dr. Nichols to watch his patients lose practically everything they have while the BWC and managed care organizations continued to thrive. In a way, it was a kind of torture for him, something that became more acute when a scandal unfolded within the BWC.

On a Tuesday night in June 2005, US Representative Marcy Kaptur informed her colleagues on the floor of the House of Representatives about a problem. She said, "There is a major political scandal that is unfolding in the state of Ohio." Ms. Kaptur told her colleagues the Ohio Bureau of Workers' Compensation had lost $215 million from an extremely risky investment.

Ms. Kaptur placed the blame directly on Governor Taft and said, "The governor of our state has permitted millions and millions of dollars of workers' money from the Ohio Workers' Compensation Fund to be invested in high risk investments."

The BWC acknowledged the loss shortly after Ms. Kaptur made her statement, but had known about the loss for a significant period of time. The huge loss did not come as a surprise for Governor Taft because he had known about the loss in October of 2004, but said nothing. With the presidential elections in November of that year, Taft had a good reason to remain silent. Ohio was up for grabs in the election and the race between Kerry and Bush tightened considerably in the final weeks of the campaign. Ohio had become a pivotal state for both candidates.

If voters had discovered that $215 million dollars were missing from the BWC and benefited the Republican Party, it would have proved fatal for Bush in Ohio, especially if the money laundering allegations were correct. The national press, disgruntled Republicans and the Kerry camp would have pushed the story to the forefront.

A review of the records showed that in 1998 the BWC hired MDL Capital Management, located in Pittsburgh. Over a course of several years, the state of Ohio had invested $355 million in a long-bond fund managed by MDL. In 2003, MDL approached the BWC and offered a proposal that consisted of the creation of what was then termed an active duration fund. The fund was supposedly intended to operate as a hedge fund. Normally a hedge fund is designed for an exclusive and very wealthy set of investors and has exemptions from regulations that control derivative contracts, short selling and fee structures. The BWC agreed to the proposal.

The bureau invested hundreds of millions of dollars but within a short period of time the hedge fund, which was based in Bermuda, augered into the ground and took with it the money the state invested.

James Conrad, the BWC administrator chief executive, discovered the loss in the MDL fund on September 27, 2004. Now the presidential campaign was getting very tight and the any information released about the scandal would have a significant impact on the election.

According to the Toledo Blade, "James McLean, the bureau's chief investment officer, told Mr. Conrad in a conference call that when he wanted to 'tighten the screws' on MDL, chief financial officer Terrence Gasper had told him that Mr. Conrad had given permission to 'give MDL a break.'"[29]

Although Conrad denied the call, Gasper said he also discussed the loss with George Forbes, appointed to the BWC oversight commission by then governor George Voinovich. Research has revealed that the tapestry that veils the BWC and the state government from outside inspection is carefully constructed to conceal an intricate pattern of corruption utilizing a network of cronyism on par with that found in organized crime. Just one of countless examples is Forbes' daughter, Mildred, who was hired by MDL in 2001.

The Ohio Ethics Commission and the Inspector General launched an investigation into the BWC investment practices. Two days after the hedge fund loss was revealed, the bureau asked MDL to shut down the fund.

Still Taft's office fought to keep the lid on this scandal, but something else surfaced that put damage control into panic mode.

A malodorous breeze of another scandal wafted through the restricted passageways of the BWC and the state house that would kill Bush's chances of carrying Ohio. Governor Taft's aides scrambled to contain the problem until the election results were final. The breeze mixed with dark smoke from a brushfire lit by Thomas Noe, an influential and powerful member of the Republican Party.

---

[29] Toledo Blade: June 19, 2005 article by James Drew and Steve Eder

Noe was the chairmen of the Bush-Cheney campaign in northwest Ohio. Allegations surfaced accusing him of giving the Bush campaign laundered money. According to the Toledo Blade, "The Bureau also became a political money making machine for Mr. Voinovich, Mr. Taft and the Ohio Republican Party – a tool to help them finance elections with multimillion dollar bureau contracts going to political contributors and political supporters such as Tom Noe."[30]

Where did Noe get the money?

In 1996, Ohio's General Assembly made some major changes that allowed the BWC to invest in stocks, real estate and rare coins. The bureau had only been able to invest in bonds before the changes went into effect. Without hesitation, the bureau embraced those changes, and so did some powerful people who had strong ambitions, people like Tom Noe and his political allies.

Over a period of several years, originating in 1998, the BWC gave Noe $50 million to create a rare coin fund. After a review of the investment in 2000, Noe's management of the fund disturbed Keith Elliot, the head of internal audits for the BWC. He said the management practices of Noe "could potentially expose both the BWC and the fund managers to adverse public scrutiny regarding the appropriate use of state funds."

Like dogs, top people at the BWC and powerful Republican politicos tried to bury the bone. In 2003, glaring problems with the fund started to emerge and some high-ranking state officials did not like what they saw.

Two state owned coins with a value of $300,000 went missing supposedly from the mail. Another group of coins estimated to be 119 in all, and valued at $93,000 were found missing after the fund's Colorado ancillary group performed an audit. The records show that Noe overlooked informing Colorado authorities about the missing coins and the loss was not made public until the Toledo Blade's stories were published. There was another prime example of the kind of fraud the bureau and Noe practiced. Money meant for injured workers somehow made it directly into Noe's pocket.

An anonymous source within Ohio law enforcement told the Toledo Blade that Noe sold one coin for $1. The value of the coin at the time was $100,000. That money could have paid for medically necessary treatments for injured workers like Bill Durst or Perry Marteney. Instead, injured workers were robbed blind and political coffers were filled.

Apparently, Noe had given money to fellow Republicans so they could donate to the Bush campaign and as news leaked out, an investigation was launched to see if any campaign contribution laws had been broken. Noe was thorough. He donated to practically every noted Republican in Ohio. Noe gave money to five out of seven Ohio Supreme Court justices, Ohio governors,

---

[30] Toledo Blade: December 17, 2006 article by Steve Eder and James Drew

senators and President Bush. Noe even gave Arnold Schwarzenegger $10,000 for a special fund. H. Douglas Talbott, a high-ranking aide to Governor Taft, was given $39,000 to buy a house in Louisiana. Noe also loaned $500,000 of BWC money to a man that used rare comic books as collateral.

Noe took care of his wife Bernadette's business as well. The attorney general's office had given her law firm contracts worth thousands of dollars. Her firm was to collect the debt on those contracts on behalf of the state.

Covering all of his bases, he assured himself that his friends in power would not chop down the money tree and would do anything they could to keep the theft from the public.

Fortunately for the Republican Party, the person heading the investigation was Gregory White, the US Attorney for the Northern District of Ohio, a Bush appointee. White said any announcement about the allegations and the investigation could not be made before November 2, 2004, which happened to be Election Day.

Senator Voinovich, Governor Taft and other high-ranking Republicans worried about their future. The pressure from the Bush camp was also influential in trying to keep the scandals from the public.

As word spread, some of Noe's cohorts worried about the money he had given them as reimbursement for contributions they made to the Bush campaign. A few of them did return the money. The Bush/Cheney campaign returned $4000 out of the $100,000 it received and Governor Taft returned the money given to him. However, Governor Schwarzenegger has not returned any of the $10,000 given to him by Noe.

The real explosion of Tom Noe's dealings and the major losses in investments were kept out of the news before the election, and the Republicans hoped that the final tallies would be in before Ohioans found out had happened. However, another controversy erupted on Election Day that sent the Republicans into hyper-drive, as they did what they could for the Bush campaign.

The election was dire for both political parties and charges of voter fraud erupted with unnerving frequency. Some voter registrations were denied in Ohio because they were not submitted on the proper weight paper and serious allegations about voter suppression were leveled at those in power.

Representative Dennis Kucinich, a Democrat from the 10th district said, "Dirty tricks across the state, including phony letters from Boards of Elections telling people that their registration through some Democratic activist groups were invalid and that Kerry voters were to report on Wednesday [the day after the election] because of massive voter turnout. Phone calls to voters giving them erroneous polling information were also common."[31]

---

[31] November 10, 2004-A *Note on the Presidential Election in Ohio*
http://www,commondreams.org/views04/1110-31.htm

Was this just a desperate attempt to take a shot at the Republicans? In Michigan, it seems the Republicans set out to suppress voters. A Michigan state legislator, Republican John Pappageorge said, "If we do not suppress the Detroit vote, we're going to have a tough time in this election."[32] Although Pappageorge said his remarks were taken out of context, the Republicans in Ohio agreed with his position and the record shows that a large suppression of votes did indeed happen in Ohio.

According to a Democratic National Committee study that was conducted in 2005, the issue of long lines and a wait of several hours to vote ended in at least 3% of the voters abstaining from the election.

There was also a significant problem in voting machine availability. A disparity between some precincts existed where there were an abundance of machines in some areas and a lack of machines in another.

Double voter registrations were also discovered in Ohio. The Cleveland Plain Dealer reported that 27,000 voters were registered in both Ohio and in Florida. According to the articles, supposedly 400 of those voters cast ballots in both states.[33]

The hanging chads were also an issue for Ohio in the 2004 election. Punch card ballots were still used and 90,000 ballots supposedly did not include a Presidential vote because of hanging chads or indecision on the part of the voter.

To add to the voting controversy, Representative Stephanie Tubbs Jones of Ohio and Senator Barbara Boxer filed a Congressional objection to the certification of Ohio's Electoral College Votes on January 6, 2005. This was only the second time that an entire electoral delegation was objected to in the history of the US. Both the Senate and the House nixed the objection, but the objection underscored the amount of corruption taking place in Ohio.[34]

It also underscores the lengths the Republican bastion in Ohio was willing to go to ensure they were victorious and could keep the money flowing into their war chests from the BWC.

While the Bush campaign, the top politicos of Ohio, Tom Noe and his friends benefited from Workers' Compensation money, workers like Diane Ferro were on the verge of losing everything they had because the bureau and their managed care organizations did not want to spend money to treat them. Evidence strongly suggests that the bureau feels that injured workers are riskier investments than rare coins and hedge funds.

---

[32] Associated Press July 21, 2004 Democrats Blast GOP Lawmakers "Suppress The Detroit Vote' Remark
[33] Plain Dealer October 31, 2004 Voters Double-Dip in Ohio, Fla. Scott Hansen, Dave Davis, Julie Carr Smyth
[34] Senator Boxer's Press Release on January 6, 2005: Statement On Her Objection to the Certification of Ohio's Electoral Vote. http://boxer.senate.gov

In Ms. Ferro's case, a simple accident at work catapulted her into a catastrophic collision in 2004 with the BWC and her managed care organization, Sheakley, which is the third worst managed care organization in total claims litigated and in cost of appeals to employers.

Ms. Ferro was 55 and had been active all of her life. She played and coached soccer was in business with her husband until they divorced and ran a daycare in her home for over twenty-seven years. One day she tripped over a doorstop at work, fell and hurt her ankle. The original diagnosis was the push button response, a sprain and strain of her right ankle. The doctors ordered X-rays, but no MRIs were performed. The months following the accident proved it was something more significant. Her injury was so bad that in order to get around, Ms. Ferro had to walk on the top of her foot. The doctors who saw her clamped onto the sprain diagnosis like terriers. After all of her years as an athlete, Ms. Ferro knew it was something more, but could not get the help she needed. One day after the frustration became too much, she told her doctor that she might as well drive her car through the intersection, and kill herself.

She went home in despair. Before she knew it, seven squad cars, one motorcycle officer, paramedics and the fire department descended upon her home. The doctor had reported she was suicidal and emergency services wasted no time in getting there. Ms. Ferro's boyfriend came home in the midst of the flurry thinking the worst.

Eventually, she gave in and went to the hospital where she talked to a counselor. The counselor recognized that Ms. Ferro just needed to get treatment for her injuries and that she would not kill herself. Ms. Ferro had a relative that had committed suicide and she knew what that would do to her family.

After over a year from her original injury, she asked for a new doctor, who finally ordered an MRI that proved she was telling the truth about her ankle. She had torn ligaments, torn cartilage, ripped tendons and her anterior cruciate ligament was torn in her right knee. In addition, there were loose bodies around the knee itself.

The doctor said she needed surgery and was appalled that her condition was so bad. Knee surgery had to wait until the ankle surgery was healed and she had recuperated sufficiently to handle another operation.

In a cast up to her hip for several weeks and then in an immobilizer for another eighteen weeks, Ms. Ferro had to adjust to the life-changing injury. Not able to do the things she did prior to her accident, she found the rehabilitative process extremely difficult. The pain she felt was quite severe. She went from a person who rarely took an aspirin to taking several medications throughout the day. The frustration of dealing with the BWC and Sheakley made the recovery worse and her emotions quickly frayed. It only made matters worse when a representative of Sheakley told Ms. Ferro that the pain was all in her imagination.

Sheakley fought her every painful step and denied treatments that could help her. Not able to work, Ms. Ferro's finances fell apart. She tried to do what she could to survive including selling jewelry to make ends meet. After falling behind in her mortgage payments, her home went into foreclosure and she was forced to find another place to live. Without adequate income, her choices were bleak. The one place she could afford was a termite-infested cottage no bigger than a double car garage and in a dangerous part of town. Most of the windows were boarded up and the wiring was over a hundred years old. Ms. Ferro's water lines were hooked up with her landlady's house and often the water would run out.

Unable to pay all of her bills, her son helped her with utility payments and did what he could, but Ms. Ferro was nearly destroyed at the prospect of relying on her son for financial help. The BWC cutoff her payments because they claimed she was overpaid. The only allowance she got was $24 every two weeks. That was it. Unable to work, unable to walk for any distance and unable to stand, she was desperate.

She began selling her plasma twice a week. Since the amount of money paid for plasma was determined by a person's weight, Ms. Ferro stuffed coins in her pockets so that she could get more money. This proved detrimental to her health. She started passing out after visiting the plasma bank and she was cutoff as a donor. Ms. Ferro informed Sheakley that she had to sell plasma and the response was underwhelming. Her caseworker told her she should not do that. Then Ms. Ferro asked how she could survive on $24 every other week and there was no response. Sheakley did not care. The only thing they told her was, "We're doing all we can."

While Tom Noe parlayed BWC money into a sizable fortune for himself, and sold rare coins to finance his interests, Ms. Ferro said she "Sold everything but myself to get by."

She was given a chance to go through Vocational Rehabilitation. Placed in a computer-training program, Ms. Ferro had high hopes that she could find a good position once Voc Rehab was complete. However, she quickly discovered the classes were not what she expected. Given tapes to listen to, she was placed before a computer and left on her own. Not used to this kind of instruction, Ms. Ferro found it difficult to learn the programs. When she asked her instructor if he would help her through the process, he told her to listen to the tapes. Frustrated at not being able to understand the lessons, she tried to get her instructor to sit down with her and explain a few things. The instructor was paid $300 per week for each student in the class and according to Ms. Ferro; he was more than willing to help the male students, but not the women.

After tough days in class and in pain, she found it overwhelming and cried every day. She finally got help from a caseworker in creating a resume and was entered into a four-week training program at Cox Cable in Akron. The training could result in getting a job offer and Ms. Ferro hoped things would change.

She had to drive a long way to the training and at the time, gas prices were high. Living on $24 every two weeks, there was not much left over for necessities like food. An independent Vocational Rehabilitation counselor, Kathy Trumm, of Korcare, came to her aid and took her grocery shopping. She told Ms. Ferro to buy whatever she needed. Ms. Ferro later said of Ms. Trumm that she was an angel that really came to her rescue when Sheakley, the BWC and others would not.

The training process was especially difficult because she would not get paid until she finished the four-week program. She did her best, but she was faced with large obstacles at Cox. In order to go on a break, she had to climb 50 stairs on crutches and then go down the stairs again and this was required several times per day. It proved to be too much and Ms. Ferro reluctantly had to quit. Her ankle and leg just could not sustain the effort and neither could her finances.

Still in a great deal of pain, and an ankle that was not stable, Ms. Ferro tried to get some relief. A caseworker at Sheakley told her that she was healed, but that was not the case. In fact, the ankle and the tissues around the ankle showed significant atrophy.

The regular BWC pattern of pushing an injured worker into pain management continued in Ms. Ferro's case and she eventually was put into a pain management program and given medication that would help, but it came after quite a battle.

During the process, Kathy Trumm guided Ms. Ferro and informed her of her rights to see other doctors in hopes of getting better treatment. Until Ms. Trumm stepped in, Ms. Ferro said, "I didn't know I had the right to be a human being." Records show clearly that injured workers are not treated like human beings by the BWC or managed care organizations. The injured worker is viewed as something far less and the only value they have is the amount of money their case will bring into the agencies.

For politicians and the unscrupulous people working within the system that is the only important thing. The interconnection and peer pressure is so strong that very few workers within the system go against the party line. Those who dare to change the status quo are punished, pressured and eventually fired.

In fact, evidence of BWC tactics easily suggests that intimidation and blackmail have been used to preserve the status quo regardless of who gets hurt.

Dr. Nichols and Kathy Trumm have worked tirelessly for the injured workers, who come to them for help. They inform them of their rights and how to get through the BWC and obtain the necessary treatments. They have been faced with an inordinate amount of pressure and so have their injured workers because they bucked the system repeatedly.

In Ms. Trumm's case, she found that the intensity of the pressure became much more pronounced. Her computer files were hacked and the names of her files were changed, but she was undeterred. Finding some irregularities in her bank account, she started missing some money. Checks started bouncing when she knew very well that there had been enough money in the account to cover them. Owning an independent Voc-Rehab company made her an instant target of the BWC and her strong sense of right and wrong guaranteed she would not play according to their rules.

Her clients were told directly that they would not get the assistance they need, and as with Ms. Ferro, every request became a battle.

In reviewing the actions of the BWC and its affiliated MCOs, it is clear that there is an orchestrated effort to follow a set protocol, which ensures that very little is done for injured workers. Policies of the BWC and MCOs are skewed towards their financial end, abandoning common decency and their original mission of assisting the injured worker. Yes, some injured workers do receive help, treatment and retraining, but the majority enter a war zone from which a healthy escape is nearly impossible. Those that do get out, like Diane Ferro, are blessed to have made it out alive.

She has been able to get her knee operation and has gotten a part-time job with Dr. Keith Ungar, an Akron chiropractor. However, more surgery is necessary in the near future due to the lack of correct and prompt treatment immediately following her accident.

Although Tom Noe was convicted and sentenced to eighteen years in prison for his crimes, Ms. Ferro has been sentenced to a lifetime of pain and disability. While Noe used BWC money to buy three luxury homes, a boat and paid off thousands of dollars of personal debt, like many victimized by BWC, Ms. Ferro lost her home and had to sell personal belongings in order to eat.

Governor Taft pleaded "no contest" to four misdemeanor ethics charges involving his actions with Tom Noe and acquired the dubious honor of being the only Ohio governor convicted of a crime; he can walk away with his health. Ms. Ferro does not have that luxury nor has she regained her dignity, which was stripped by the BWC.

While some people lost their jobs because of their involvement in the scandal, they have the ability to work full-time in other positions. Ms. Ferro will never be able to be fully employed.

Even though the investment scandal was in 2004, the BWC and the current governor, Ted Strickland, have learned nothing. Injured workers are still abused on a daily basis, while the corruption continues within the BWC and the MCOs.

The Ohio Auditor's office spent an additional $645,000 of taxpayer money in their investigation of these crimes, an investigation that might not have been launched at all if The Blade had not gone public with its investigation.

The Republicans might have been chased out of office, but it is still business as usual for this well-oiled, well organized money-making machine; until someone has the courage to tear it down, injured workers will continue to die, some will commit suicide, some will become crippled and will develop insidious depressions, not from their work, but from the crimes of those in power. As has been noted, this number is in the thousands, documented in one state alone.

This investigation has uncovered the root problem that is at the core of the BWC and MCOs. Much larger entities and more powerful players well beyond Ohio planted the seeds of greed and fraud. When the seeds sprouted, the thorns and weeds flourished in these crime-riddled environments and successfully choked most of the remaining decency and morality in the workforce. As they grew unabated, they became more powerful. Those groups not only have used this system to obtain huge profits, but they have also used the system as a laboratory experiment, where injured workers are their guinea pigs.

Without ending their reign of terror, these groups will manipulate the rest of the country much in the same way and our rights as human beings will be increasingly nullified.

CHAPTER SIX
RACKETEERING OHIO STYLE

In doing interviews for this book, there seemed to be several commonalities which surfaced throughout their course. Whether the interview involved an expert or an injured worker, invariably when the discussion turned to the BWC and the MCOs and how they operate, the subject of organized crime was mentioned. Interviewees suggested the likelihood that organized crime was behind or at the very least connected in some way to the bureau and its managed care organizations.

When people hear the term "organized crime," most think immediately of the mafia or La Cosa Nostra; but there are other elements that must be considered when dealing with organized crime. As we have seen lately in the financial crisis, some of the biggest criminals operate outside of a Mafioso family environment, but that does not make their crimes less heinous.

Within La Cosa Nostra there are rules that must be obeyed and certain lines that are never crossed. However, with a different kind of crime syndicate, fewer rules are in play and consequently almost anything goes. Due to the lack of rules, there has been a tendency in some of the criminal structures to function on an every man or woman for himself/herself basis, although their ultimate goals might be shared. At times, this can lead to critical infighting.

In studying the inner workings of the bureau, it is obvious that the agency operates in a disorderly fashion verging on pandemonium. Only a few people really know what is actually happening within the agency in any given department. This dysfunction benefits the perpetrators who take advantage of the system no matter where their allegiance lies or who is calling the shots.

Let us look at how organized crime is defined to determine whether or not it applies to what is happening within the BWC and the MCOs.

According to the California Commission on Organized Crime, "Organized crime... is a technique of violence, intimidation and corruption which, in default of effective law enforcement, can be successfully applied, by those sufficiently unscrupulous, to any business or industry which produces large profits. The underlying motive ... is always to secure and hold a monopoly in some activity which will produce large profits. Sometimes the basic business is illegal... Sometimes the basic activity is legal and is a racket only because of the violence and corruption with which the business has become permeated."[35]

There is no question that this definition applies to the bureau and some of its affiliated MCOs. A monopoly does exist. Any outside entities that are perceived as threats are targeted through various tactics that could be deemed illegal such as coercion, intimidation and personal threats in order to ensure that huge profits will continue. The actions within the BWC also fall under other definitions of organized crime.

The US Comptroller General has referred to it this way: "'Organized Crime' refers to those self-perpetuating, structured and disciplined associations of individuals or groups, combined together for the purpose of obtaining monetary or commercial gains or profits, wholly or in part by illegal means, while protecting their activities through a pattern of graft and corruption."[36]

On the federal level, "The FBI defines organized crime as any group having some manner of a formalized structure and whose primary objective is to obtain money through illegal activities. Such groups maintain their position through the use of actual or threatened violence, corrupt public officials, graft, or extortion, and generally have a significant impact on the people in their locales, region, or the country as a whole."[37]

When considering the maneuverings within the BWC, it is apparent that the system has all the criteria to be attractive to criminal elements, whether they are white collar criminals associated to people in power or an organized crime family. Vast sums of money are at stake, as already mentioned, which only enhances the temptations.

A legitimate business or state agency like the BWC is chartered to operate above the law to help injured workers and employers, but it is obvious that criminals have used the BWC for financial gain in an organized and manipulative way. The lack of oversight on the part of the BWC regarding

---

[35] Special Crime Study Commission on Organized Crime, 1953: 11

[36] U.S. Comptroller General, 1981: 10

[37] Federal Bureau of Investigation website:
http://www.fbi.gov/hq/cid/orgcrime/glossary.htm

their investments and the funds in general has given criminals a nurturing environment and allowed them to operate virtually unfettered.

The existence of criminal activity within the bureau is present in several forms. Intimidation is used against injured workers; doctors like Dr. Nichols who refuse to be part of the corruption are targeted and third-party vocational rehabilitation companies that voice objections about the BWC's methods and the lack of treatment for injured workers.

Kathy Trumm has experienced sharp intimidation tactics, both verbally and financially from those within the bureau. Her clients have been warned by the bureau not to seek her services and if they do, the injured workers have been told they will not get the help they need. Ms. Trumm fought back and weathered much of the intimidation process and had to file Cease and Desist orders. The bureau, however, kept changing the rules. When it came to submitting paperwork for injured workers, companies like Ms. Trumm's KorCare were given a three strike you're out policy, which meant that the outside companies helping injured workers could only submit three late reports before they lost their affiliation with the BWC. Kathy Trumm's efficiency in filing reports was questioned on several occasions, but she was able to prove she submitted the necessary paperwork on time. The bureau has since dispensed with its three-strike rule. People who know Kathy Trumm well have said that her integrity and her honesty are incomparable, yet the bureau continues to coerce her.

Like Dr. Nichols, Ms. Trumm has had people in black SUVs watching her house. It seems that most people that stand up against the illegal methods of the BWC are normally followed and intimidated. The bureau's tactics resemble those employed by gangsters and confirms the fact that a criminal element is well entrenched within the agency. The bureau's contempt for the law grows unchecked because of the tremendous lack of supervision and the amazing lack of curiosity on the part of law enforcement. Governors have repeatedly given a pass to the bureau and its questionable way of doing business because it is in their best interest -- in doing so it gives the impression that they are calling the shots within the bureau. While some politicians have called for investigations, returned campaign contributions and distanced themselves from the BWC, the fact is that the governors have not severed their ties nor have they been healed of the dependency on BWC dollars.

The very nature of the BWC and its propensity to engage in questionable and immoral activities even after Coingate and other investment scandals along with the complicity of politicians confirms the presence of a crucial factor in determining the existence of organized crime within the agency. That factor is "self-perpetuating criminal conspiracy for power, profit, utilizing fear and corruption and seeking immunity from the law."[38]

---

[38] Rhodes, 1984, 4. Definition of organized crime.

The BWC's conspiracies for profit will not work without people and institutions willing to facilitate their plans, and of course, there has to be something in it for them. There are many people who benefit from the investment money the bureau seems to throw at investment houses and banks. From individuals to corporations, millions of dollars grease the wheels of several entities that would like to remain silent partners with the BWC.

From a business standpoint, it is understandable that the BWC would want to invest the inordinate amount of money it has to ensure that there is a decent return on investments and to grow its assets. Although those investments have not always been wise, it appears that is less important to the bureau than the need for those investments to be politically and corporately expedient. Those dubious investments create a strong alliance with the private sector and in the process grow tentacles that put a death grip on all opposition, another key element for the basis of organized crime.

Due to the large amount of money that is handled by the BWC and its investment and deposit potential, Ohio banks have benefited greatly from their association with the bureau. Their alliance can help in other ways as well.

One case in particular is the relationship between the bureau and Allegiant Asset Management. The bureau had given Allegiant, an extremely politically connected investment company, millions of dollars to invest on its behalf. Like its previous investments, the bureau lost $71 million with Allegiant's management. According the bureau, $60 million of those losses were because of poor management decisions on the part of Allegiant.

Opponents of Governor Taft wanted to know why it took the disclosure of other investment scandals to announce this most recent loss. According to Allegiant, the bureau was kept appraised of the fund's performance, however, the bureau did not agree. Although the fund was bleeding severely, nothing was done until the losses became public.

To appreciate why the bureau was reluctant to do anything, we can look at the connections Allegiant had with National City Bank. First, National City Bank of Cleveland at the time owned Allegiant Asset Management wholly. The bank and its employees were quite politically active and financially committed to Ohio politicians.

The bank's political action committee and its employees gave more than $1 million to Ohio politicians over the course of several years since 1990. The bulk of the money went into the pockets of Republican candidates, although some Democrats benefited. The BWC's cash cow gave birth and eventually a small but formidable herd started to grow. The Republican wranglers, like former Governor Taft, were more than willing to remain silent about it. Taft's campaigns got $61,975 from National City contributions. During his gubernatorial campaigns, Senator Voinovich received $50,737 from National City.

State Senator Mark Dann said that Allegiant's losses really offered more proof those political contributors prejudiced the BWC's financial transactions. Dann stated, "There were extraordinarily well-connected campaign contributors at National City Bank. For years, [the bureau] just allowed the losses to mount without taking any action against their political benefactors."[39]

Naturally, banks are necessary for state governments to handle public funds and National City was quick to point out that state funds are deposited based on bids. What National City failed to say is that it would not remain completely neutral in their business dealings, particularly as they related to the public or more precisely, how they related to opponents of the BWC. Dr. Nichols and Kathy Trumm, who were vocal about the malfeasance and fraud within the bureau, found that National City could be a daunting adversary even though they were customers of the bank.

After waging several battles with the BWC, Ms. Trumm found that funds were missing from her bank accounts and checks started to bounce from both her business and personal accounts. Being a savvy businesswoman, she knew how to handle money and was well aware that there were enough funds deposited into her account to more than cover any expenditure. Funds mysteriously disappeared for over two years. She still does not know what happened to the money. Eventually she changed banks and has not had similar problems. Recalling what National City did, Ms. Trumm said, "They almost broke me."

Considering National City and Allegiant Asset Management were beholden to the BWC, and not about to go against a significant investor, it is quite likely that National City allegedly did the BWC's bidding when it came to intimidating Ms. Trumm and manipulating her bank accounts.

The shenanigans were also directed at Dr. Nichols. During the time the BWC was investigating him and delaying his payments, Dr. Nichols had to do something to try to save his practice. He wanted to restructure some loans and went to National City Bank for help.

He spoke with a loan officer who recommended that Dr. Nichols consolidate his loans and have one smaller payment, which would help him while he waited for the BWC payments. He was given the impression it was a done deal and was told to check back within a couple of weeks. Dr. Nichols contacted the bank and was told it would be a little longer, but things were fine with the loan. As he waited, things got rougher financially for the Nichols family, but he remained patient. After two months, Nichols called the bank and was shocked to learn that National City would not do the loan. Due to the bank's stall tactics, he took a sizable financial hit and lost his home and car. It

---

[39] July 8, 2005 Toledo Blade Article: Firm fired after losing $71M from BWC; officials blame fund managers By Steve Eder, Joshua Boak, and Blade Staff Writers

appeared that the BWC was successful in stopping Nichols for a time, but he did not give up and neither did Kathy Trumm.

The interactions of the BWC with National City Bank demonstrate that the bureau has encouraged or strongly influenced its allies to engage in its efforts to stop any opposition that would ultimately expose its plans even if that meant ruining their opponents. When depositors place tens or hundreds of millions of dollars in various banks, the banks do not wish to risk losing that business and will generally acquiesce to their demands.

Managed care organizations are drawn to the big dollars that the BWC doles out and they play a significant role in keeping the profit margins high, which can impact how injured workers are treated, if they are treated at all. Since 1997, MCOs have received in excess of $1.374 billion and in turn have donated over $610,000 to political campaigns. As soon as MCOs were allowed to get into the workers' compensation field to facilitate the BWC's administration of claims, competition has been intense in this lucrative milieu.

Ohio employers fall prey to the ravenous MCOs, whose hunger can foster unethical practices in signing the finite number of employers. It is not uncommon for MCOs to get creative when it comes to adding clients, especially in open enrollment periods. They can get quite imaginative when it comes to signing clients because the more clients they have, the more injured workers they have and that means more money is paid them by the Bureau of Workers' Compensation.

One such MCO, 1-888-OhioComp has been known to be extremely forceful in getting employers to sign with them. The company is run by Jason Lucarelli, and has developed a questionable reputation in Ohio and particularly with other managed care organizations. Lucarelli is the son of Samuel G. Lucarelli the head of a powerful Cleveland family with ties to organized crime.

In 1989, Sam G. Lucarelli was implicated in a loan sharking and illegal gambling venture located in Cleveland, was convicted and served time in prison. Although Jason Lucarelli runs 1-888-OhioComp that did not stop Sam from allegedly making a curious phone call to an owner of a third-party administrator company, whose clients are companies involved with workers' compensation cases.

Bonnie Fraser, the president of Actu-Comp claimed that she got a call from Sam G. Lucarelli. According to Ms. Fraser, Lucarelli asked her if she was interested in sending her clients to his son's company, 1-888-OhioComp, for which she would receive ten percent of the money those clients brought into the company from the Bureau of Workers' Compensation.

Ms. Fraser further stated that Lucarelli allegedly offered to pay her in either quarterly or yearly payments. Ohio state regulations forbid MCOs from offering any remuneration to third-party administrators for referrals. According to the bureau, such kickbacks would result in the MCO losing its contract with the BWC and becoming decertified.

Allegations of kickbacks are not new to the bureau and dozens of cases have been investigated since 2004. The bureau also receives over 6,000 allegations every year involving workers and their injuries that are also handled by their investigative unit. Most of the kickback allegations were unfounded supposedly, but the investigations were not conducted with real enthusiasm, but rather with the bureau's usual tepidity.

Only one allegation was considered to have merit and the managed care organization was neither decertified, nor did it lose its contract. Instead, it could not accept any new employers for a three-month period.

Ms. Fraser's allegation against Lucarelli went nowhere. In fact, there were no records at the BWC to indicate that investigators even talked to Lucarelli. The records did show that investigators had a conversation with his son, who claimed that neither he nor his father had offered Ms. Fraser money. Stamping the allegation as unsubstantiated, the BWC closed the case.

Upon learning of the decision, Ms. Fraser stated, "Apparently, they don't want to investigate this for some reason. They don't want to turn over the rocks, and that is not a good thing."[40]

As in numerous other incidents, the bureau has been concerned with political ramifications in nearly every move it makes. Handling the allegations against Lucarelli was no exception.

The Ohio Money Tree and other campaign contribution records show that the Lucarelli family, the executives of their company and the chief executives of other MCOs have donated hundreds of thousands of dollars to Ohio campaigns for years.

In 2006, the tables seemed to turn on the Lucarellis, who informed the bureau that GatesMcDonald Health Plus allegedly offered a kickback to the city of Cleveland, if it signed with them.

The Lucarellis had gone after the city of Cleveland's business nearly at the inception of 1-888-OhioComp and took exception to the supposed move by GatesMcDonald. The mayor's office quickly denied that any managed care organization had offered a kickback, and that ended the BWC's special investigation. The investigators never contacted GatesMcDonald.

There have been other charges of wrongdoing and kickbacks and after brief investigations, some lasting only a few days; the allegations are rubber-stamped "unfounded" and immediately closed.

The Lucarellis benefited greatly from the BWC. From 1997 through 2006, 1-888-OhioComp received $29 million for managing injured worker cases. Of course, they were not the only ones to benefit from the bureau's money; the Lucarellis donated substantial sums to several influential Ohio candidates.

Governor Taft received $27,000. Governor Strickland received Lucarelli contributions totaling $23,825 for his congressional campaign. Ohio Attorney

---

[40] Toledo Blade December 17, 2006 article by Steve Eder and James Drew

General Jim Petro received $7,000, which would have dampened any investigations that could have been launched against 1-888-OhioComp. A long list of mayors and county supervisors as well as the Republican Party had to send Thank-You cards to the Lucarellis for their generosity. In total, the Lucarellis and executives of their companies donated $218,000 to various campaigns.

The Lucarellis have also been known to use powers of persuasion, especially when millions of dollars are at stake. One source stated that the bidding process of the MCOs was not bad until 1-888-OhioComp opened shop. The sources stated that city and county governments made decisions about which MCOs, they would sign with and the atmosphere was free from coercion. However, when 1-888-OhioComp entered the equation, decisions were no longer based on the performance of individual MCOs, but were politically based. In fact, if an elected public administrator did not sign with the Lucarelli company, that person would find that the Lucarellis would put up their own candidate to run against them in the next election.

Jason Lucarelli admits that his company wines and dines prospective clients, but according to him, public employers are not courted the same way. If 1-888-OhioComp's competitors are telling the truth, the Lucarellis allegedly have used intimidation in their bid to sign as many employers as possible during open enrollment. Whatever the company is doing seems to be working because it is the fastest growing managed care organization in Ohio. While most MCOs disagree with how the public sector has subsequently decided on which MCO will represent their agency or government, the bureau finds nothing wrong with how the Lucarellis do business.

Federal agents watched 1-888-OhioComp and have investigated some of its employees after allegations surfaced about a supposed association between Cuyahoga County Auditor Frank Russo and the Lucarelli company in 2008. Russo's son, Vince, was employed as a consultant for 1-888-OhioComp and helped to recruit clients for the company. Competitors of the Lucarellis were concerned that improprieties were involved in the recruitment process. Allegations arose because 1-888-OhioComp handles claims for most of the public employers in Cuyahoga County.

According to subpoenas that were filed in Cuyahoga County, investigators seemed to think that the Lucarelli company was allegedly part of the overall corruption of the county government. Frank Russo's association with the Lucarellis troubled investigators. Not only were the people at 1-888-OhioComp well-connected politically, but Russo's employees were also well-placed politicos, who lobbied on behalf of the Lucarelli firm. The Plain Dealer stated that Russo had 283 employees and of those, 93 held political rank. Fourteen of those employees were either current or former members of boards of education and city councils. One mayor who took exception to the Lucarellis big increase in signing public employers said that the lobbying tactics were questionable and that the County Commissioner, Jimmy Dimora and Frank Russo pushed 1-888-OhioComp on those employers.

The mayor of Maple Heights, Jeff Lansky, claimed that Dimora and Russo asked the Lucarellis to fundraisers and supposedly introduced them to various mayors of Cuyahoga County who had the ultimate decision in deciding on MCOs for their government. Lansky further stated that 29 public agencies switched to 1-888-OhioComp from 2002 through 2004. He was certain that the governments switched to the Lucarelli company because of the introductions by Russo and Dimora.

"All that was done because Lucarelli – and he had a lot of help from Russo and Dimora – pressured a lot of mayors in Cuyahoga County, calling on I.O.U.s and personal favors and things like that," Lansky stated.[41]

Maria Smith, spokesperson for the Bureau of Workers' Compensation did not respond to questions about 1-888-OhioComp's alleged unethical business tactics and why the company had not been decertified or sanctioned for its purported misconduct according to BWC standards.

Politicians are reluctant to go against the Lucarellis either because the family has contributed heavily to their campaigns or perhaps because of alleged strong-arm tactics used by the Lucarellis, tactics not dissimilar to those used in loan-sharking.

Sharon Ray, Medina County Commissioner spoke to the Plain Dealer about intense pressure she received from Tony Capretta, who at the time was a Brunswick councilman. She accused Capretta of allegedly threatening her. After Medina County turned down 1-888-OhioComp's overtures, Ray said that Capretta told her, "The boys aren't very happy with you. We came and you didn't take care of my friends. They think I should run against you."

While the BWC turned a blind eye to the unethical tactics of 1-888-OhioComp, other MCOs like UniversityComp yelled foul. However, all of its protests fell on deaf ears at the bureau; Joe Catalongo, rumored to be friend of the Lucarellis, eventually bought out the company.

A problem surfaced within the bureau where one of its employees was doing work for 1-888-OhioComp and other former BWC employees on state time and using the bureau's resources. It came to the attention of the Inspector General's office that Kevin Rearick was running his graphic design company during his employment with the BWC. He supplied printed materials to his clients that were printed using the State Printing and Mail services. According to the Inspector General's remarks dated September 17, 2008, "Rearick was performing this work, directly or indirectly, for clients that were either owned or managed by or had employed seven former BWC employees."

---

[41] November 30, 2008 Plain Dealer article, *Auditor Frank Russo's links to workers comp firm investigated*, by Rachel Dissel and James Ewinger

One of those clients was 1-888-OhioComp. Emails obtained through this investigation showed that Dan Neubert, who runs the day-to-day operations at 1-888-OhioComp, had Rearick doing printing for the company. It was not known if Neubert knew that Rearick was using state equipment for his business.

Rearick did have access to the BWC computers and as such posed a security threat. An email dated March 28, 2008 from Kevin Rearick to Pam Hiles, who was communicating to him for Dan Neubert at 1-888-OhioComp, suggested that he might be under surveillance. Rearick stated in the email, "Nope on board of director meeting days I'm here the whole day so I won't be able to do anything until after 5. I'm not even taking my drive to work these days to remove any allegations that anyone may have."[42]

If Rearick brought his hard drive or thumb drive into work, he or anyone else at the bureau had the capability to copy BWC information. Through the course of the investigation for the book, it has been learned that the BWC has a secret file level that is used to enter and to communicate information about injured workers, MCOs, IME doctors and so forth. Anyone having access to that level could harvest critical data for themselves or other interested parties.

According to Karen Conrad, the president of the International Association of Rehabilitation Professionals and former president of CareWorks, a customer service specialist or CSS has the ability to access the secret file level. Further, a team clerk working in concert with the CSS pulls together pertinent information that is sent to IME doctors. Therefore, the clerk has the ability to withhold information that would help an injured worker during a medical exam. Doctors might be influenced by the information or the lack of it when deciding on whether an injured worker is disabled or in need of treatment.

Ms. Conrad said that IME doctors do not have direct access to the secret level of files unless a CSS gives them the password to access them or if the doctor goes to the BWC personally, where they could obtain the information.

The control of information is pivotal in understanding how the bureau operates in regards to the injured worker and how the doctors working for the bureau interact with them. By picking and choosing information to send to review doctors, the BWC can significantly impact the results of any medical exams and/or hearings that take place as a result of benefits being denied. Such control ensures that the bureau can contain its costs and maximize profits.

A prime example of criminal activity present within the BWC, which involves the manipulation of crucial data, is the case of injured worker, Lewis "Rex" Whan. This case clearly demonstrates the organized nature of crime within this government agency.

---

[42] Evidence taken from Inspector General's investigation into Kevin Rearick dated September 17, 2008

Mr. Whan, a Navy veteran who served on the USS Forrestal in 1962 during the Cuba blockade, was doing well in 1981. He had a good job and a wonderful family. He was married with ten children, whom he adored. One day during his shift at Akro, Incorporated, he was working on a cure press binding carpet to rubber backing. The top of the clamshell press began to slam down rather than close slowly and Mr. Whan had to catch the lid, which weighed somewhere between 75 and 100 pounds. This had to be done repeatedly throughout his shift. Mr. Whan was paid by the piece and had to keep the pace up in order to make enough money. Before the end of his shift, Mr. Whan was in intense pain and could hardly walk. His foreman sent him home.

By morning, he was much worse and had to go to the doctor. He tried to get into his truck to drive, but could not manage it. His wife had to drive him. When he saw the doctor, the Workers' Compensation doctor asked him to bend over. Mr. Whan could not do it because of the severe pain.

That did not satisfy the doctor and he screamed at Mr. Whan to bend over, but he could not do it. Still the doctor screamed at him to cooperate. Finally, Mrs. Whan could not take it, and shouted, "You son of a bitch, he can't bend over!" Even though Mr. Whan could hardly move at that point, the doctor said he was fine and could go back to work.

Remaining in horrible pain over the weekend, his wife's grandfather suggested that Mr. Whan see Dr. Meyers for another opinion. After Dr. Meyers had evaluated Mr. Whan, he told him he was unable to go back to work for a year. He had suffered a herniated disc made worse by substandard treatment from the BWC doctor. The Whans had to live without his paycheck for a year. If it had not been for their savings, they would have drowned financially.

The treatment course of events was the BWC's norm and Mr. Whan had to do much of his recuperation on his own. He did finally make it back to work, but his back was never the same. Suffering a great deal of pain, Mr. Whan resumed his duties, but it nearly drove him into the ground.

For eight years, Mr. Whan suffered through his job. In 1989, he was on a ladder about fifteen feet from the ground doing inventory. Two people worked below him on the ground as they counted the rubber sheets used for car mats. Suddenly, a tow motor was being driven in their direction. Unfortunately, the tow motor did not have any brakes and by the time the driver saw the ladder it was too late. The driver tried to veer into pallets to slow down and a domino effect hit.

Mr. Whan saw it coming and grabbed onto the rung of the shelving overhead just as the ladder was knocked out from under him. He hung on as long as he could, but eventually fell to the ground. His neck, shoulder and thoracic spine were hurt.

Mr. Whan did get some treatments and benefits from the BWC, but unfortunately, he could not return to his full workload at Akro, Incorporated.

He was placed on light duty for a time, then the company told him that there was no job description for light duty and he was let go until he could return to his original position.

Over the course of a few years, it was established that Mr. Whan had suffered permanent disability rated at 112% by the BWC standards, but then something strange happened with his file. Certain records were erased and his physical impairment suddenly dropped to 87%. Of course, his benefits dropped as well. Mr. Whan had no medical improvement in his condition to warrant the change, the approved disability records just vanished.

At a hearing, his attorney, Jonathan Goodman, called the BWC on what happened. The bureau's attorney said that no one had complained before, indicating that there was a precedent for this kind of illegal activity. Mr. Goodman told the attorney that you just could not go into an injured worker's file and delete arbitrarily pertinent information on their medical records. Unbelievably, Mr. Whan lost the hearing and now has only one more avenue left to him.

As with Perry Marteney and thousands of others, an IME doctor asked Mr. Whan what made the pain worse. He responded, "Living." Mr. Whan remembering his service during the Bay of Pigs and the Cuban Missile crisis said, "I thought I was fighting the enemy, but I know now the enemy is right here in this country." Like Perry Marteney, Mr. Whan sits at home in terrible pain and stares at his gun cabinet and thinks of ending it all. Without relief and without justice, he wants to stop unbelievable suffering. If he does, the bureau's bottom line will improve, and no doubt bonus bucks will be distributed for getting another injured worker off the books. The State of Ohio would lose yet another worker, which it deems disposable.

Of course, the bureau could not continue its behavior without showing some modicum of benevolence to some injured workers whom the BWC can use as "success" stories. This is another aspect of true organized crime, in that a legal business is run on several different levels to mask its criminal operations.

Governors appoint the director at the Bureau and as long as there is a lack of control and checks and balances in place, the bureau will continue to operate outside the law, squashing opponents and injured workers with reckless abandon. The American political process and the enormous amount of money it takes to run campaigns creates a need for entities like the bureau to fuel those campaigns with dollars that should be used for the injured workers.

The "genetic makeup" of the BWC not only promotes corruption from within, but also from outside sources that have a vested interest in controlling the cash flow.

Hearing Officers within the system also perpetuate the criminal atmosphere by accepting doctor opinions that are based on lies and on seldom performed exams by those doctors. By accepting those file reviews that doctors mail to the bureau, they are engaging in the fraud. Specifically, wire and mail fraud occurs when doctors knowingly send falsified reports through the mail or by wire for which they are remunerated. The hearing officers are accessories to those crimes, but it is the injured worker who is treated like the criminal.

Additionally, the BWC could not continue to carry out its diabolical exploitation of the vast majority of injured workers without the help of criminal doctors. Many of these doctors have worked out a system that abuses the injured worker with independent medical exams, while they do the BWC's bidding. How far will doctors go to commit fraud? Videotape evidence, which will be covered in the next chapter, proves that some of these doctors will stop at nothing to get the job done for the BWC and to stake a claim in the bureau's goldmine.

CHAPTER SEVEN
PROSTITUTE DOCTORS AND
THEIR CRIMES

Many things stand out when it comes to the overwhelming evidence of the criminal behavior within the Bureau of Workers' Compensation's regime. One of the major factors is the extent to which people will go to make money at the expense of the injured worker. When reviewing the videotaped evidence and the falsified documentation, it is appalling to discover the deliberate prostitution present within the system. Some doctors describe their colleagues who take part in this corruption as "whores" because they falsify their medical reports, do not give correct or thorough exams and base their evaluations on a 97% denial rate for fear they will lose their BWC certification status and incredible profits.

By comparing various videotapes of independent medical exams, it became clear that the methodology was the same. It did not matter whether the doctors were medical doctors or chiropractors. The lack of standards in those examinations became the dubious "standard" by which hearings officers determined which injured workers would be allowed treatment and those who would be denied.

Certainly, there are guidelines established by AMA or Chiropractic associations about how specific exams should be conducted, but it is up to the individual doctor to use them. Dr. Nichols thinks that it is imperative for doctors to use the guidelines. He said, "The doctor would take the higher ground/standard when evaluating an IW [injured worker] especially when you consider everything that is at risk."

There also seems to be a pattern of how fraud is committed by doctors that practice outside the legal framework. The Industrial Commission does have a manual for Disability Evaluator Panel doctors to use, but according to Dr. Nichols and from gathered evidence, it is plain that the doctors are not using it. Some of these renegade doctors determine results by pulling numbers and findings out of thin air. A review of the medical reports submitted to the BWC and MCOs indicate that the doctors submitted false information and were paid handsomely for it.

For instance, we can compare independent medical exams done by BWC approved doctors to see how the specific doctors break the law. In Mr. Whan's case, his IME doctor, Edward Waldo, D.C. had a polished routine and an ebullient façade used to make the injured worker feel as though he was on their side, as he did with Mr. Whan. Allegedly, the doctor was falsifying his reports and changing or eliminating Mr. Whan's own words from the record. Mr. Whan gave thorough and honest answers about his injuries and the pain and numbness he had. He was consistent throughout the years with what he told his doctors and what he told Dr. Waldo during his independent medical exam.

Dr. Waldo failed to ask open-ended questions and in fact, led Mr. Whan in his answers. He even chose words for Mr. Whan to describe his condition in a multiple-choice format without giving Mr. Whan the opportunity to go into detail about his pain and injuries.

Dr. Waldo seemed to listen to Mr. Whan and wrote down notes as the exam progressed. His solicitousness verged on that of a used car salesman when he asked Mr. Whan a bevy of questions that were contained in the BWC paperwork. However, the answers he charted did not reflect what Mr. Whan actually said.

Further, during the exam Dr. Waldo used a goniometer[43] to determine the range of motion in his arms. According to AMA guidelines, to evaluate permanent impairment, a dual inclinometer[44] should be used, not the goniometer, in order to accurately assess the real range of motion. When it came to measuring the range of motion in Mr. Whan's lower back, the video shows that Dr. Waldo had no measuring device in his hands, but he did write down a capricious number as if he had truly measured the range of motion. Mr. Whan was denied an MRI based on Dr. Waldo's report and he subsequently filed a criminal complaint on the hearing officer, Gary J. Frame, who used the false information in making his decision to deny the claim.

The complaint dated, September 14, 2009 stated, "As an employee of the State of Ohio, District Hearing Officer Gary J. Frame, in his capacity to preside as a Staff Hearing Officer in workers' compensation claims, in particular claim

---

[43] Oxford Dictionary: An instrument for the precise measurement of angles.
[44] Oxford Dictionary: A device for measuring the angle of inclination of something esp. from the horizontal.

number 81-31926 and 89-67003, was required according to 4123.10[45] to investigate in such manner as to ascertain my substantial rights and to carry out justly the spirit of such sections."

Regarding Dr. Waldo's exam and his findings, Mr. Whan further stated in his complaint, that "I clearly had right sided symptoms according to the "Patient Pain Drawing." Dr. Waldo lied about the MRI request being directed at "left-sided pain and tenderness." Dr. Waldo also diagnosed me with "Left Brachial Radiculitis"[46] and instructed me on home recommendations for my pain. Dr. Waldo fabricated the ranges of motion of my neck, both shoulders and my low back. He also fabricated many other parts of his "examination" as well as "history/complaints."

Mr. Whan asserts that Dr. Waldo was paid for the exam and committed not only workers' compensation fraud, but also wire/mail fraud, a Federal offense, when he mailed the falsified document to the BWC.

The hearing officer, in order to make a determination in Mr. Whan's case, used Dr. Waldo's allegedly erroneous and fabricated findings. Although a lawyer represented Mr. Whan and submitted that the exam was not valid, Mr. Frame chose to base his decision on Dr. Waldo's flawed findings ignoring any evidence presented by Mr. Whan. He denied the claim for Dr. Nichols' prescribed diagnostic test.

Mr. Whan's criminal complaint stated that Gary Frame, a licensed attorney, "exhibits neglect of duty and in violation of § 124.34[47] to consider any

---

[45] 4123.10 Industrial commission not bound by rules of evidence.
The industrial commission shall not be bound by the usual common law or statutory rules of evidence or by any technical or formal rules of procedure, other than as provided in sections 4123.01 to 4123.94, inclusive, of the Revised Code, but may make an investigation in such manner as in its judgment is best calculated to ascertain the substantial rights of the parties and to carry out justly the spirit of such sections.

Effective Date: 11-02-1959

[46] Radiculitis is the inflammation of the nerves that carry signals from the spine to the shoulder, arm and hands.
[47] (A) The tenure of every officer or employee in the classified service of the state and the counties, civil service townships, cities, city health districts, general health districts, and city school districts of the state, holding a position under this chapter, shall be during good behavior and efficient service. No officer or employee shall be reduced in pay or position, fined, suspended, or removed, or have the officer's or employee's longevity reduced or eliminated, except as provided in section 124.32 of the Revised Code, and for incompetency, inefficiency, dishonesty, drunkenness, immoral conduct, insubordination, discourteous treatment of the public, neglect of duty, violation of any policy or work rule of the officer's or employee's appointing authority, violation of this chapter or the rules of the director of administrative services or the commission, any other failure of good behavior, any other acts of

evidence that I had showing that the medical record submitted by the examining physician Dr. Edward Waldo was untrue and deceptive."

By basing a decision entirely on alleged falsified medical records; Frame jeopardized any integrity of the adjudicatory process, which violated the Commission and Hearing Officer Code of Conduct, R96-1-6.[48] Frame gave preferential treatment to Dr. Waldo and ignored any evidence from Mr. Whan.

Dr. Nichols believes the independent medical exam is skewed at the outset because injured workers are only seen for fifteen to twenty minutes and evaluated on pain that might be present only during that particular moment, creating a mere snapshot and overlooking the bigger picture that would reflect the injured worker's true condition. The snapshot exams are structured in favor of the evaluating doctor who zooms in on a statement the patient might have been led to make that does not focus on the whole injury. In Mr. Whan's case, Dr. Waldo seemed to purposely focus on the left side of Mr. Whan, an area not covered under allowable conditions with the BWC and thereby assuring the claim would be denied.

An IME doctor can and does override the Physician of Record or POR during a brief encounter with the injured worker even though the POR might have been following his patient for years and thus more knowledgeable about the injured worker's true medical condition. By superseding the Physician of Record's opinion, it dubs the POR as incompetent. Additionally, it casts a light on the POR that they are in league with someone who is a malingerer or faker, when in most cases that is not the case.

One former IME doctor, that prefers to remain anonymous, stated, "The cold hard truth is that Managed Care will not pay these kinds of fees to render a favorable judgment. However, much as they deny it, IMEs have already been bought. I have always accepted a Managed Care company's request to act as an IME. As soon as it became clear that on occasion I might indeed support the injured worker's diagnosis, such requests abruptly stopped coming my way."

Mr. Whan had other symptoms and pain that he detailed in the "Patient Pain Drawing," but not once during the videotaped exam did Dr. Waldo discuss those symptoms with him. He shifted the entire exam away from any

---

misfeasance, malfeasance, or nonfeasance in office, or conviction of a felony. The denial of a one-time pay supplement or a bonus to an officer or employee is not a reduction in pay for purposes of this section.

[48] WHEREAS, Chapter 4121-15 of the Ohio Administrative Code, the Industrial Commission Code of Ethics, provides, in Section 4121-15-03(G), that the intent of the Industrial Commission's Code of Ethics is "that employees avoid any action... which result[s] in or create[s] the appearance of: (1) using public office for private gain, or (2) giving preferential treatment to any person, entity or group:"

allowable condition and as a result, his recommendation was to deny the claim as unnecessary.

In a sense, the injured worker gives the examining doctor a deposition, which under the Industrial Commission is considered fact. However, in reality, the answers charted by the doctor might not reflect what the patient said, as was the case with Dr. Waldo. Decisions are based on blemished medical exams many of which contain fictitious results.

Independent Medical Examiners are instructed on how to handle the exams and what they need to do to achieve the desired results, which are frequent denials of claims. The injured worker has no such coaching and is left on his own to face a system that is rigged at the outset.

This is true not only for injured workers within a workers' compensation environment, but any employee or insured person that applies for disability benefits. Insurance companies operate in the same way as the BWC and utilize doctors that are known to render desired decisions about a person's disability.

With the Industrial Commission, there is another line of defense against the injured worker and that is the hearing officer, who under no uncertain terms keeps his/her job by denying claims. The multi-level system within the BWC tips the scales in favor of the bureau and away from the injured worker even though the law states emphatically that no preferential treatment should be used in the adjudication of claims. The tremendous prejudice that exists within the hearing officers operations reflects a serial abuse of the law, which seldom is corrected. Due to the large number of people involved in dealing with the claims, the buck is passed from one person to another and no one is really held accountable for malfeasance and abuse of the law.

Gary Frame should have been reprimanded for his actions, but nothing has been done in answer to Mr. Whan's criminal complaint. The Bureau of Workers' Compensation and the Industrial Commission claim to have a low tolerance for fraud, but they turn away from any corruption taking place in their own agencies. On rare occasion, allegations of fraud have supposedly been investigated, but those cases are nominal.

Another prime example of the illicit machine that foments the corruption and fraud within the bureau is the case of Audrey Smith, an injured worker from Carrollton, Ohio. She worked for Colfor Manufacturing. Her job consisted of taking baskets of tools out of sonic washers.

The baskets are heavy and several employees had complained about trying to lift them. The job is repetitive and difficult to do. One day, Ms. Smith tried to lift a basket of tools that was particularly heavy out of the sonic washer and felt an awful burning sensation in her neck and right shoulder.

She went to her supervisor to alert him to the problem. Many company officials go on the defensive when injuries occur and Ms. Smith's injury was no exception. Her supervisor told her that an accident report had to be filed before she could leave and go to a hospital. The supervisor put the brakes on and even after prodding by Ms. Smith to get something done so she could get medical attention; it took the company five hours to get the report filled out.

No one from the company assisted her in getting to the hospital. She had to drive herself. Ms. Smith went to Aultman Hospital and one of the first things she was asked was whether or not her injury happened at work. She was checked over by the staff, but no MRI was ordered and no X-rays were taken. The doctor put her arm in a sling and sent her back to work.

Unable to work because of the pain, Ms. Smith went to see Dr. Nichols to get his opinion on her injury. He immediately took her off work and set up an MRI, which showed severe tendonitis.

During the course of her treatments, she was scheduled for an independent medical exam with Dr. Richard Kepple of North Canton, Ohio. Her brother, Bill, who brought with him Dr. Nichol's video camera to tape the examination, accompanied her to the exam.

When Dr. Kepple entered the exam room, he made it a point to mention that only a blood relative or spouse could be present for the exam and he seemed to be caught off guard by Ms. Smith's brother. Kepple was assured that Bill was indeed a blood relative and he started the exam.

Dr. Kepple asked a series of questions about her injury and the pain she experienced. Then he proceeded to measure her range of motion in her neck and her arms. As he placed the goniometer on top of Ms. Smith's head, she complained that he was pushing down too hard and it hurt her. Kepple responded that he was only trying to keep the meter in place.

He then tested the range of motion in her left arm and moved to her right arm. As he stood behind her, he moved her arm back and up and Ms. Smith asked him to stop because it hurt. Dr. Kepple kept going and something popped in her arm. The videotape showed clearly that Ms. Smith was indeed in a great deal of pain and started to cry. Kepple was unmoved and kept up with the exam. Ms. Smith told him that he hurt her, but he did not respond and did not check to see what had happened. He appeared oblivious to her complaints.

He asked her to stand up and she told him to give her a minute while she tried to compose herself and waited for the pain to subside, but it did not relent. She stood after two or three minutes and turned to finish the exam. However, she could only go through a few more tests and needed to quit. Kepple left the room because Ms. Smith was being what he considered to be uncooperative.

The video showed her right shoulder was tensed and visibly higher than the left shoulder and Ms. Smith could not move her arm. The pain was so great that she could not help but cry. Concerned, Bill called an ambulance to come to the doctor's office.

During the wait for the ambulance, not one person in Dr. Kepple's staff came in to check on her and the doctor did not return to the exam room. The ambulance arrived several minutes later and the paramedics had to assist Ms.

Smith onto the gurney. As she left the doctor's office, no one on staff said anything to her. Ms. Smith was taken out, placed in the ambulance and taken to Aultman Hospital.

At the hospital, the ER staff examined her and she told the physician's assistant that she felt like her arm was going to fall off. Ms. Smith was given two shots for the pain and something for nausea. She was sent home with two prescriptions for pain. One was Ultram 50 mg taken every 6-8 hours as need for pain and the other was Vicodin 500 mg-5mg every 6-8 hours as needed for pain for 3 days.[49] Obviously, the Emergency Room staff deemed the prescriptions necessary to help Ms. Smith with the aggravation of a previous injury brought about by the independent medical exam.

Unfortunately, Ms. Smith's trouble did not end with the visit. Her attorney, Jonathan Goodman was notified that she was to have another IME exam because Dr. Kepple would not issue a report. He claimed she would not cooperate during the exam and therefore he was unable to render an opinion. Dr. Kepple did not say that Ms. Smith was physically unable to complete the exam.

Ms. Smith went to Dr. Nichols who ordered an MRI. The results showed that she had severe tendonitis and bursitis that flared since her exam with Dr. Kepple; a condition that the BWC said was already healed.

Without being able to work and going through a divorce, Ms. Smith was in financial distress. The independent medical exam performed by Dr. Kepple complicated her recovery and delayed her return to any kind of employment. Having to go through another IME in order to get treatment and benefits stalled any forward momentum. Those unreasonable delays have not helped Ms. Smith to keep a positive attitude. The helplessness that workers feel when they need and want to work and are physically unable to is particularly stressful. With the Catch-22 process used by the BWC, workers find it nearly impossible to break the cycle.

Some IME doctors have their exams down to a science of how to maximize profits in the least amount of time, ignoring overwhelmed injured workers. An outrageous example of pimping the system is the case of Byron Melville, whose injuries from work and his recovery process typify the flawed system that the BWC allows to prosper and paints a hideous portrait of the medical profession.

Mr. Melville worked for Colfor Manufacturing as a press operator and sorted parts for cars and motorcycles. During the course of his day on July 10, 2006, he had to move a four-foot by four-foot rubber mat that weighed about twenty pounds and that had a heavy grinder sitting on it. As he pulled the mat behind him, the mat got caught in a hole in the floor and the grinder fell on the

---

[49] Aultman Hospital Emergency Department prescriptions for Audrey Smith

mat, jerking his right arm to the floor. Mr. Melville let go of the mat and tried to catch the grinder in his left hand, but was unsuccessful.

He went to Aultman Hospital and was given an injection for the pain, along with other medications and returned to work with restrictions. Mr. Melville was not supposed to use his right arm. However, every job at Colfor was a two-handed job. Colfor did not accommodate his work needs. He found that he had no choice but to do what he could, even if that meant aggravating his injury. Due to the continued abuse to his arm, Mr. Melville saw a physician who took him off work.

On May 9, 2007, Mr. Melville had a mandatory IME exam with Prasanna Soni, MD, who is an orthopedic surgeon. He showed up for the examination on time, and was accompanied by his friend, Jefferson, who carried a bag containing Dr. Nichols video camera. He signed in and filled out paperwork, but the doctor kept him waiting for nearly an hour. He was then taken to an examining room where he waited for a few minutes before Dr. Soni arrived.

Dr. Soni entered the exam room, but left the door open. The doctor asked Mr. Melville some questions over the course of merely forty-five seconds. Then Dr. Soni started the physical exam. He looked at Mr. Melville's right arm and elbow and then the left arm and elbow. His evaluation lasted thirty-eight seconds. He asked Mr. Melville a few more questions that took approximately one minute and fifteen seconds. Then he asked Mr. Melville to stand, put his arms up and put them behind his back, as if he were being handcuffed. These motions were terribly painful to Mr. Melville who had been advised previously by his physician not to raise his arm. Those tests took thirty-two seconds. Dr. Soni handed Mr. Melville some paperwork for the receptionist and concluded the exam. The total time of the exam was four minutes and two seconds. The hands-on exam was barely a minute in duration.

Although the total length of time Dr. Soni spent with Mr. Melville was slightly over four minutes, he billed the BWC $450 for an hour of his time. Further, Dr. Soni used no instruments to measure Mr. Melville's ranges of motion, did not check his reflexes and did not examine his right elbow, which was also injured.

However, Dr. Soni filed a fraudulent report based on his quasi exam and determined that Mr. Melville had no abnormal problems in his shoulder and elbow, and was not experiencing any tenderness in the injured sites, contrary to Mr. Melville's complaints and findings from other physicians. Soni stated that Mr. Melville reached maximum medical improvement and could return to work without restrictions. Yet, Mr. Melville left the exam in extreme pain. Dr. Soni was paid for his fraudulent report and Mr. Melville was back at square one.

Mr. Melville went to John N. Reister, MD, who on August 31, 2007 performed an arthroscopy of his right shoulder and decompressed Mr.

Melville's shoulder and he also released the lateral epicondyle[50] of his right elbow. This surgery would not have been performed had there not been sufficient evidence to indicate the surgery was necessary for Mr. Melville. Dr. Soni's fraudulent report should have been shot down by the BWC, but it was not.

Mr. Melville contacted the fraud unit and informed them what had transpired during Dr. Soni's IME with him. According to audiotapes, the bureau's employee was cordial to Mr. Melville, and took down his information, but apparently nothing was done to investigate the allegations of fraud against Dr. Soni.

This is not an isolated incident with either the bureau's paltry response or with fraudulent doctors. Mr. Melville was faced with another IME exam and this time it was with Dr. Oscar F. Sterle, MD, an independent medical consultant certified by the BWC. Again, Mr. Melville went armed with a video camera and had a friend go with him as a witness.

Dr. Sterle's nurse, Cathy, took down Mr. Melville's medical history, but did so in a rushed, confrontational manner. She rolled her eyes when Mr. Melville could not answer her questions quickly enough and was impatient and rude with him throughout the entire process. She set the tone for exam with Dr. Sterle.

When Dr. Sterle entered the room, he asked Mr. Melville a series of questions about his injury and medical history. When Mr. Melville could not remember specifics quickly enough or could not recall the answers, Dr. Sterle got annoyed and starting shouting at Mr. Melville. Being frustrated, Mr. Melville shouted back, stating he honestly could not remember the answer. Sterle terminated the exam and stormed out of the exam room without examining him. With the antidepressant medication Mr. Melville was on, it is no wonder that he had trouble recalling the minutiae that Sterle wanted. The doctor should have been well versed in what antidepressants can do to a person's memory and taken a more charitable approach in his evaluation.

When it came to filing his report, Dr. Sterle stated that he conducted an exam and his nurse collected a medical history from Mr. Melville. He also mentioned that the exam was terminated because of the verbal abuse aimed at him by the injured worker.[51]

It is important to note that independent medical exam doctors do not have a doctor-patient relationship, but rather one of a supposedly unprejudiced, independent doctor evaluating an injured worker. Ideally, the IME doctors

---

[50] Lateral epicondylitis, is a painful condition of the elbow caused by overuse. The forearm muscles and tendons become damaged from overuse — repeating the same motions again and again. This leads to pain and tenderness on the outside of the elbow. Orthoinfo.aaos.org

[51] Dr. Sterle's Medical Report dated September 26, 2008 and sent to CIME Management, Dublin Ohio

should truly be independent and not give preferential treatment to the agency requesting the exam over the injured worker. However, given that the bureau, employer or managed care organization pays for the services, it can and does sway the doctor, especially if that doctor wants a steady stream of injured worker exams and income.

A case in Virginia sent an interesting message to IME doctors that might injure or harm an examinee during an evaluation. While the doctor-patient relationship is not rooted in the normal sense during an IME exam, it is possible for an IME doctor to be sued for malpractice.

The case was Harris v. Kreutzer and was heard by the Virginia Supreme Court, which considered whether or not a person can have a private cause of action against a doctor who was ordered to perform and independent medical examination, like those working for the BWC.[52]

Ms. Harris alleged that she had an automobile accident that caused her a traumatic brain injury in 1991. She had an independent exam performed on her by Jeffrey Kreutzer after which she purportedly suffered a deterioration in her previous conditions that were post traumatic stress following a robbery and the traumatic brain injury. Ms. Harris claimed in the suit that Kreutzer deliberately was abusive to her during the course of the examination and she suffered emotional trauma in addition to the supposed deterioration of her prior conditions, which she asserts that he knew about them and thereby committing a tort of intentionally inflicting emotional "distress."

The Supreme Court held that "the consensual nature of the physician/patient relationship may be express or implied." That decision left open in part the question of malpractice since Dr. Kreutzer agreed to perform the examination.

The court ruled that any malpractice had to occur during the examination itself and not from a report that would be filed by the examining doctor. Ms. Harris claimed that Kreutzer went out of his way to inflict emotional stress on her. Although the court did not rule on the specific incidents, it did rule that malpractice could exist under the relationship of an IME doctor and the examinee. The implications in the future are great for doctors that consider taking on IME assignments. Other states will no doubt follow suit in instances such as these, which would clearly remove the imbalance that exists within the confines of IME exams and would afford some protection and redress for patients like Audrey Smith and Byron Melville. Doctors would no longer be able to act with impunity.

Some injured workers do not wait for something to happen before they take action, but when injured workers try to protect themselves, retaliation is swift. One of Dr. Nichols' patients, Tishya Albright, decided to be open and up front with Paul Bartos, MD who was scheduled to give her an independent

---

[52] Harris v. Kreutzer, 271 Va. 188 (2006)

medical exam. Bartos broke the rules before Ms. Albright ever made it into his office for the exam. A physician that is scheduled to perform an IME cannot have contact with the injured worker prior to the exam. Bartos clearly crossed the line by sending Ms. Albright forms to be filled out ahead of her scheduled IME.

Uncomfortable with the situation, Ms. Albright went to the exam with her brother who carried a video camera in plain view. She felt it was her right and within the law to videotape the exam. Dr. Bartos thought otherwise and said that no video cameras or recording devices were allowed in the exam. In part, that is true. The guidelines, though, are referring to physicians taping the exams, not the patient. Her brother had a copy of the Ohio Revised Code with him and informed Dr. Bartos that Tishya had the right to intercept any communication involved with the exam and to video record the full examination. Bartos declined and a stalemate occurred.

Bartos then filed a report with the BWC stating that the IME was called off because Ms. Albright and her brother were videotaping the offices, the certificates on the wall, the sign-in sheet and other patients. The videotape shows that Tishya was taped signing in, the doctors' certificates on the wall were taped, but no patients were taped. A person behind the desk approached them and said that Dr. Bartos was not part of their company and only rented space from them for his exams and that the company did not want to get in the middle of things. Their representative did not say that the taping must be stopped. In essence, the company gave its assent to Ms. Albright and her brother by not asking them to stop the taping or asking them to leave.

When asked why she let Dr. Bartos know ahead of time that she would be recording the exam, she said it was important for her to be upfront. Obviously Dr. Bartos did not agree and the results of the complaint he filed resulted in Ms. Albright's claim being suspended.

With three herniated discs in her lower back and living with considerable pain, the news was not good for this young wife and mother of two small children. In many ways, Ms. Albright was fortunate that her husband was able to take up the slack with the financial crisis, but it was a highly unnecessary situation.

Other problems arise for injured workers when IME doctors are in collusion with the bureau. Often there are unwarranted physical exams ordered or the injured worker is pushed into strenuous exercise that only harms him/her and needlessly lengthens recovery or makes it impossible.

There are blatant violations of ethics on the part of doctors that give independent medical exams, especially when their examinations result in the further injury of the worker. No person should have to worry that they will be placed in danger during a physical examination, but that is exactly what is happening currently throughout the country.

Recourse for injured workers that are harmed during an IME is practically non-existent. Most lawyers that are approached to handle these cases brought to them by injured workers will not take the case without at least $10,000 up front a sum beyond most injured workers, whereas the bureau, the MCOs and the prostitute doctors have deep pockets and a team of lawyers that could drag the case out ad nauseam.

Therefore, injured workers have no power of redress. After further investigation, that appears to be the intent behind the BWC's actions.

Additional methods are used to insure that the injured worker is portrayed in the worst possible way, which shifts the burden of responsibility away from the bureau and the corrupt doctors dropping it on the injured worker, who is in no condition to take on the behemoth system.

One of the surest methods used by the aberrant medical community is to question the emotional and mental stability of the injured worker, even to the extent of making the worker's families question whether or not the injuries, pains and complaints are not just something in the injured worker's head. When that happens, an insidious despair can creep in often leading to the injured worker's suicide.

Many doctors within the system that have an established record of denials focus on undermining the injured worker's credibility and they do this at the very beginning of their contact with the injured worker. That immediately makes any claims the injured worker makes about their injuries and pain suspect. If there is an inkling of depression in the injured worker's history, even if it was several years prior to the work injury, that gives the IME doctor the ammunition necessary to shoot down that particular claim. If there was no prior psychopathology, the doctors zero in on any psychological signs of depression or mental imbalance despite the fact that any anomalous psychological factors could be the psychological sequelae from the injury itself.

It is amazing that doctors that only see an injured worker for a brief period of time, often less than twenty minutes, and who have no particular expertise in diagnosing complicated psychological disorders can assess the injured worker's true emotional and mental state. Further, it is more surprising that IME doctors can cavalierly override psychiatrists and psychologists who spend substantial time with the injured worker and have issued a battery of tests in reaching their educated diagnoses. By accepting opinions of the IME doctors less qualified to render professional psychological assessments, the BWC and the Industrial Commission are engaging in prejudicial behavior aimed at debunking the injured worker's case and depriving them of benefits and justice.

Nevertheless, that is the mechanism is employed by doctors, making anything a worker says suspect. Any complaints about injuries and pain are therefore dismissed as being all in the injured worker's head. Clearly, these so called experts try to lord it over those "less educated" and use their position to further their own goals even if they have to commit fraud to do it. Once these experts dub the injured workers as malingerers or fakers, any credibility the worker might have had either within the system or within their family is often destroyed. When a psychiatric diagnosis is attached to the injured worker, the nature of the claim changes and it also changes the benefits a worker receives. Requests for treatment will be denied because the injuries might now be deemed outside the boundaries of allowable conditions because the worker can be considered a hypochondriac. The bureau might place the worker into a vocational rehabilitation program, but the necessary treatments for the original injury will be denied. Again, this is an enormous victory for the bureau and the MCOs. It is also another victory for the doctors that tag the injured worker with false diagnoses.

By signing falsified medical reports, these doctors sign away what's left of the injured worker's life. They relegate the injured worker to financial and emotional ruin leaving emotional scars that seldom heal this side of the grave.

These doctors chuck science for the so-called bureaucratic greater good, but they also chuck the truth and in doing so christen themselves charlatans and bureau whores. While these doctors cash their checks for their ignoble deeds and their prostitutions, injured workers have to subsist on the crumbs of a tarnished and broken system. Once proud, hard-working people, the injured workers are thrown into a caste to rot in a world not of their own making and from which there is no escape. The system as it stands now is rigged. Doctors are paid to render a predetermined judgment about the treatments for injured workers. The answer 97% of the time is "No." The system is neither fair nor licit, but unless this powerful machine is stopped, countless lives will continue to be ruined. As a national health care system gets closer to reality, so does the likelihood that millions will face this outcome.

Dr. Nichols felt strongly that videotaping corrupt doctors in action would result in major changes made throughout the system. He called the Industrial Commission and fraud investigators in the bureau and asked whether or not videotaped evidence showing that a doctor falsified his/her exam would be sufficient evidence to prove fraud. One investigator thought that would certainly help to launch an investigation into the examining doctor's reports and exams and that the evidence should be considered by hearings officers.

In an email from G. K. Johnson from the legal department at the bureau. He said, "This is in response to our discussion in respect to question #4 in your correspondence. As I stated, I am not aware of any bureau policy that states what type of evidence (i.e. audio, video, oral etc.) is to be considered relevant evidence. Relevant evidence is any evidence which tends to prove or disprove the existence [of] a fact that is necessary to make a determination of an issue; the form in which the evidence should be given, does not affect its relevancy. While the bureau personnel charged with deciding the issue being presented have discretion to determine whether any evidence submitted is relevant, that determination should not be based on the evidence's form.

Have the BWC and the Industrial Commission used Dr. Nichols' videotaped evidence? No. Without acknowledging the existence of evidence, without even viewing the evidence, a Hearings Officer could hardly give a just or equitable decision in an injured worker's claim dispute and the crimes of the doctors never see the light of day.

CHAPTER EIGHT
LESS THAN HUMAN

Without a doubt, the bureau and the managed care organizations are a major part of the assault against injured workers, but self-insured employers are also a vital component in this brutal war. When it comes to taking responsibility and helping the injured workers, some self-insured companies make the BWC look like an amateur in its abuse. In fact, if we look at the statistics from around the country regarding self-insured employers, they have a history of pushing their employees to the depths of despair, destroying their lives and leaving what is left to the vultures.

Some self-insured employers will go to great lengths to defame and to destroy their employees, many of whom have been with them over ten years and have given them quality work during their tenure. Often the largest and most financially secure companies are the very ones that are the worst offenders when it comes to taking care of sick or injured workers.

When these companies hire new employees, they dazzle the recruits with glowing promises of benefits, pensions, and health and disability insurance touting their responsibility and dedication to each employee. However, when someone is in need of those benefits, the company takes off its mask and exposes the true and hideous face that lies beneath. Workers are shocked at the bipolar behavior of their once beloved employer.

Such was the case with a man we will call John Doe, who worked for Coca Cola as a delivery driver/merchandiser. Mr. Doe, 34, married with two small sons, loved his job and was rated as one of the best drivers and employees in his territory. He was so happy with his job that he could not think of doing anything else the rest of his life. A former All-Ohio football and baseball star in high school, and a veteran of the first Gulf War, Mr. Doe was in good shape and took care of himself. He coached his young sons in sports and was extremely active.

On March 29, 2006, he was pulling a load of Coke cases up a curb, which weighed approximately 200 pounds, when he felt a jabbing pain in his right hip and in his right leg. In intense pain, Mr. Doe notified his supervisor of the situation according to Coca Cola protocol. The supervisor was two hours away and asked him to finish out the day. When Mr. Doe finally got medical attention, he had a five-minute exam with a doctor through Work, Health and Safety for Coca Cola. The doctor diagnosed him with a back strain. He was given 800 mg. of Ibuprofen as needed for the pain. No X-rays were ordered and the examining doctor put him on light duty.

According to Mr. Doe, light duty at Coca Cola was comprised of anything the company could get you to do. They put him to work painting and cleaning walls, which consisted or scrubbing them with brushes. It was very difficult for him because the scrubbing motion exacerbated his pain level. It got so bad that he had to sit on a stool and try to do his work.

Other factors arose that made the light duty extremely difficult for him. Fellow employees would taunt him and so did some of his supervisors. At this point, Mr. Doe was taking as many as six 800 mg. of Ibuprofen in order to work, but he knew something was not right with his back. He went to his boss and told him that the pain was making the work impossible. He sent him back to see L. Bruce Hensley DO, at Work, Health and Safety.

Hensley is not highly regarded by some of his patients or by some of the companies that have utilized his office for drug tests because he allegedly has made some questionable diagnoses without proper testing. Supposedly Hensley gave Mr. Doe a perfunctory exam. He wrote a prescription for Vicodin, which Mr. Doe took four to six times per day. After two and a half weeks, he finally had X-Rays taken. Mr. Doe also asked that an MRI be done and Hensley told him, "You are faking."

Still on light duty and unable to resume his driving for Coca Cola, Mr. Doe was receiving 20-30% less pay and the repercussions hit his family hard. Finally, he had an MRI ordered to check his lower back. He was told the results of the MRI showed nothing out of the ordinary. Yet, Mr. Doe was still in considerable pain, but was told to work through it because it was nothing more than a simple strain. He was assured that nothing was wrong with his back. That relieved his mind, but not the pain. He did what he could and tried to work through the pain, but it was not getting any better, in fact working made it much worse. Desperate to improve and to get back to work, he asked his boss if he could have two weeks' vacation to see if he could and his boss agreed.

Mr. Doe spent two weeks on the couch applying ice to his hip and back. After returning from vacation, he was released to full duty, but he had to have a helper for two weeks. Unfortunately, he only got the help for one day.

He started having jabbing pain in his right buttock and after two weeks back on the job, his hamstring started to bother him and he developed tingling in the foot. Out of necessity, he resumed taking Ibuprofen, but the pain continued to worsen. He informed his boss, who told him to keep working. By this time, pain radiated down his right leg and the severity was so terrible he could no longer drive. Mr. Doe called his boss who eventually came and got him. He was taken back to the Dr. Hensley. The doctor told Mr. Doe that he pulled his hamstring and wrapped his right thigh with an Ace Wrap bandage, but did not prescribe any medication.

At this point, Mr. Doe had to take handfuls of Ibuprofen for it to have any impact on his pain and he was unable to work. He knew that Dr. Hensley was wrong about his condition, but he did not know if he could see someone else because of Coca Cola's policy of sending their injured workers to Work, Health and Safety. Sedgwick, the MCO for Coca Cola informed Mr. Doe that he did have the right to see another doctor.

This time, Paul Welch, MD who specialized in orthopedics, saw Mr. Doe, and told him the difficulty was in his back. Dr. Welch showed him the same MRI used by Dr. Hensley and pointed to the L5 spinal area. According to Dr. Welch, Mr. Doe suffered from a herniated disc and degeneration at L5-S1. The Coca Cola doctor had lied to him about there being nothing wrong. Meanwhile, by resuming his work, Mr. Doe further injured his back. Like the BWC that used undue influence in getting their doctors to fabricate a diagnosis in the Bill Durst case, Coca Cola made sure the initial diagnosis of a sprain/strain was the only diagnosis Dr. Hensley would render.

Coca Cola proudly boasts on their website, "Our employees are the heart and soul of The Coca-Cola Company and help make us a special part of people's lives. For more than 120 years, Coca-Cola employees have led our success by living and working with a consistent set of ideals as we seek to benefit and refresh everyone who is touched by our business. This basic proposition of our business is simple, solid and timeless."[53]

Yet, in direct contradiction of their "basic proposition," Coca Cola attacked Mr. Doe, his credibility and destroyed his life. To ensure the job was complete, they hired a team of lawyers to shut down Mr. Doe anyway they could, and they used any means necessary to achieve their goal. The legal team was able to delay any treatments, payments to doctors and lawyers who were helping Mr. Doe by tying up the case in countless appeals through the Industrial Commission.

The ridiculous number of appeals that Coca Cola initiated sent no warning signals to the BWC that this self-insured company might be unjustly haranguing its employee and dragging its feet when it came to paying for necessary treatments. Rather, the BWC benefited financially from the appeals process and

---

[53] http://www.thecoca-colacompany.com/careers/careers_north_america.html

if anything, the monetary awards for delaying payments to the injured worker by abusing the adjudicatory process were enormous.

Every year injured workers file 250,000 new claims with the BWC. Each issue that goes to the appeals process costs the employer $200 and is paid to the BWC through premium rates.[54] Using a conservative estimate that each claim has at least five appeals issues involving treatment disputes that are heard over the course of five years that the BWC keeps the injured worker on the books, the BWC reaps a healthy $250 million. Many cases, like those previously mentioned have dozens of appeals that must be heard. So it is very likely the BWC actually gets approximately $500 million for those 250,000 injured workers.

You do not have to be a brain surgeon to understand that the bureau has a vested interest in denying claims and in taking the appeals process to extraordinary levels because it is good business as far as they are concerned. That is why hearing officers deny so many claims and by doing so perpetuates the agonizing appeals process for the injured worker. It is not about healing the injured worker and getting them back to work, it is about greed. Coca Cola has the funds to go along with this tainted process.

Coca Cola spends over $2 billion per year in advertising touting their products, but they have forgotten how their products get into the hands of consumers. Coca Cola forgets about the men and women in the bottling plants and the drivers like John Doe who work hard to make Coca Cola what it is. To put it into perspective, employees like John Doe delivered 23.7 billion unit cases worldwide in 2008.[55]

Accidents on the job happen. Certainly Coca Cola realizes that inevitability. Mr. Doe did not intentionally hurt himself and his herniated disc proved he was no faker, but Coca Cola continued to fight him every inch of the way. One morning Mr. Doe did all he could to go to work. He got up at 4 AM and tried to get ready for work. Mr. Doe made it as far as his living room and ended up lying on the floor. He called his supervisor at Coca Cola, John Dunnington, who said, "Sorry to hear your luck," and hung up. That was it. No one from Coca Cola checked on his condition, but instead he was viewed as an enemy.

This attitude extended to Coca Cola's attorneys and how they dealt with Mr. Doe during the appeals process for his claims. On several occasions the Coca Cola attorneys belittled Mr. Doe in the presence of the hearing officers calling him a malingerer, a faker and attacked his ability to care for his family. During one hearing, the Coca Cola attorney asked him if he was driving a

---

[54] Employer Handbook for On-The-Job Injuries 2006 Edition, © 2006 NB Comp Consultants LLC
[55] http://www.thecoca-colacompany.com/ourcompany/ar/operatinggroupoverview.html

borrowed car. Mr. Doe said he was. Then the attorney asked him if his kids were on Medicaid and Food Stamps. They were. The hearing officer allowed the barrage to continue and at the end of it, Mr. Doe said he did not feel much like a man, someone who could provide the necessities for his family. He was emotionally pinned down by the badgering and could not rally against the attorney to tell him that it was because of Coca Cola's lies, mistreatment and disdain for its employees that threw him into financial ruin. Here was a Coca Cola employee and a Teamster Union steward who worked for the company for over ten years with an excellent record. He was always there for his company. When the time came that Mr. Doe needed Coca Cola to be there for him, the company ran from reciprocity. Even the Teamsters did not help Mr. Doe, perhaps because the union feared taking on the financial giant in difficult economic times.

Meanwhile, Mr. Doe's physical pain was increasing and also his emotional distress. Of course, pain medication was approved and he got Vicodin and Percocet. When necessary, he continued to use Ibuprofen. Dr. Welch wanted to give him cortisone injections to knock out the pain, but Sedgwick gave no response. It took three months for the injections to be approved. Even an IME doctor said that the injections would benefit Mr. Doe, but that did not speed Sedgwick's decision to allow the treatment.

Once Mr. Doe received approval for the shots, he found he had an even greater problem with which to contend. His first epidural injection went fairly well and he found some relief. The second injection was not as simple. The doctor could not get the needle in and ended up tapping it into the affected area. Mr. Doe developed the worst migraine he ever experienced.

The next morning when he awoke, he could not move his head or feel his arm. He called the doctor's office in extreme pain and by this time could not move his neck. There was not much that could be done for him. Apparently, the epidural injection damaged a nerve, damaging the thecal sac,[56] which increased his pain level to intolerable levels. Placed on what Dr. Nichols referred to as a "boatload" of medication, Mr. Doe had a grueling five months that consisted of unimaginable pain and powerful, debilitating headaches. At one point, he wanted to jump off a bridge.

Wanting desperately to work in order to care for his wife and family, Mr. Doe grew dangerously depressed. Coca Cola was not helpful at any time during this period. Dr. Welch recommended that he get another MRI to evaluate his current condition. Coca Cola denied the request. Although Coca Cola claimed that they want their injured workers to recover and to get back to work, Mr. Doe is a textbook case in how the company actually treats some of its employees.

---

[56] The thecal sac consists of membranous material that encases the spinal cord with the spinal fluid.

Eventually the MRI was approved, but not before the medications damaged Mr. Doe's gallbladder, and stomach. The results of the MRI were shocking. It was discovered that Mr. Doe had no disc at L5. Apparently, it had disintegrated. The only evidence the disc was ever there was a protrusion that remained. Any surgery that could help Mr. Doe was ruled out because of his young age. Dr. Nichols treated him, which got the pain level down to 7 or 8, with 10 being the worst.

Physical therapy was requested, but it was not approved. He tried to do stretching exercises, but they only made his condition worse.

During this time, Mr. Doe had three IMEs. All the exams were done by Dr. McDaniel, which represented a definite conflict of interest and a breach of protocol. An IME doctor supposedly should only see the injured worker once in a twelve-month period. The three exams also meant that there was prior contact with the injured worker, which is supposedly not allowed by BWC standards and a predisposition to the outcome of the exams. Naturally, all of McDaniel's opinions were the same. On one occasion, Dr. McDaniel did not see Mr. Doe before determining that he had reached Maximum Medical Improvement or MMI. The case went to the Industrial Commission and they upheld McDaniel's decision without considering the entire facts of the case.

It was also during this time that Mr. Doe's son had to see a specialist. When he went to get a prescription filled for his son, he found out that his prescription card was cancelled. Coca Cola gave him no warning that his benefits were cut off. Mr. Doe called Coca Cola and they said everything was all right, but he later learned that his benefits ceased.

Like many employees across the country who lose their benefits from either illness or job loss, he was offered the COBRA[57] package. Of course, the monthly premium was so high that Mr. Doe had to decide whether he wanted to pay for the insurance or feed his family and pay the mortgage. He chose to feed his family. Most COBRA monthly premiums are so high for a family of four that you could make a monthly mortgage payment on a luxury home.

With an uninviting future, Mr. Doe cried often and found himself locked in a prison of pain and frustration. He tried to make the best of it and applied for other jobs at Coca Cola, but was unsuccessful. According to Rhonda Leach, a Return to Work Specialist at Coca Cola, once an injured worker is diagnosed as reaching maximum medical improvement like Mr. Doe, the next step is to put the injured worker into Vocational Rehabilitation so that they can get better. Then the injured worker can get back to work, but not for Coca Cola. They would have to find employment elsewhere.

---

[57]

http://cobrainsurance.com/?source=google_adwd&gclid=CNWHlPDi7J0CFQ4MD Qod1z6tQQ

With the help of his attorney, Jonathan Goodman, Mr. Doe was allowed back benefits eventually, but when it came time to receive the check, that was a different matter. Sedgwick claimed the check was in the mail, but weeks later, Mr. Doe still had not received his check. Dr. Nichols tried his best to help him get that check, which would help him to provide for his family, but Nichols hit a brick wall. It took ten weeks for the check to finally arrive, but Mr. Doe was faced with another problem. All of Dr. Nichols' treatments for him were denied so that he could not get any relief from the pain he experienced.

Dr. Nichols made several calls to Sedgwick on behalf of Mr. Doe and asked their representatives how they expected him to get better and how they expected him to survive. He got no answer. Depression set in and Mr. Doe had to see a psychologist to help him through it.

Further chiropractic treatments with Dr. Nichols have been denied to Mr. Doe. However, those treatments seem to be the only treatments that alleviate some of his pain. As a result, Dr. Nichols treats Mr. Doe without charge at least once per week, although he should have more treatments. Mr. Doe does not want to take advantage of Dr. Nichols' generosity.

This case is not yet resolved and an Ohio Supreme Court battle is scheduled in the near future in anticipation that the higher court can force the Industrial Commission and Coca Cola to do their duty and award Mr. Doe the benefits to which he is entitled.

According to Jonathan Goodman, Coca Cola has done nothing illegal in handling Mr. Doe's case, but they have treated the case with an absence of morals and fairness. They have turned the disability case into a legal three-ring circus in order to avoid paying Mr. Doe for the just compensation for his injuries.

Mr. Goodman said that self-insured employers like Coca Cola could become a nightmare for the injured worker. Due to the fact that the BWC has no direct control over self-insured companies, injured workers often suffer more abuses of their rights. Self-insured companies have an inordinate amount of power and they can say "No" no matter what. Their deep pockets make it nearly impossible for injured workers like Mr. Doe to be treated fairly, especially without competent legal counsel.

Even with good attorneys, the contentious nature of the large self-insured companies like Coca Cola guarantees that the injured worker's claim will be fought for years. Many injured workers grow weary of the process and find there is no hope for justice. Without lawyers like Jonathan Goodman, sadly that is the case and certainly without doctors like Dr. Nichols, injured workers would not be able to find relief.

Mr. Doe struggles to cope with the uncertainty that has become his family's reality. The children get their clothes from Goodwill and cannot enjoy the latest video games or eat out with their friends. They also cannot enjoy the more important things like being coached by their dad in sports and being able to do things with him like they once did. The family's home came close to foreclosure and they still live month-to-month not knowing if the family will end up in a trailer. Despite the inordinate amount of stress, Mr. Doe tries to keep focused on the things that matter. He has reconciled himself to the fact that if they do end up in a trailer, at least his family will be together. Still, this is not the life Mr. Doe originally provided for his family through his employment with Coca Cola. His savings and his investments are gone. His hope in Coca Cola to make good on their "basic proposition" and to take care of him is all but vanished leaving a terrible hole where his dreams once lived. Now he looks into the eyes of his wife and children and wonders what will become of them. Struggling with suicidal thoughts on a daily basis, Mr. Doe tries to believe he will win, tries to believe that there is still some decency and justice to be found in a world that finds him expendable. Until then, he hopes and prays that when he looks into his wife's and sons' eyes, he sees the reflection of the man, the husband and the father he wants to be for them.

Smaller self-insured companies can also pose severe problems for their sick or injured workers. The family atmosphere that many smaller companies claim they enjoy is frequently found to be nothing more than a flimsy façade when an employee has an accident.

Such was the case with Kitty Schuster, a college graduate who chose to work at Colfor Manufacturing because the pay was much better than she could get working in her chosen field. Ms. Schuster needed the extra money to care for her husband who was diagnosed with COPD, congestive heart failure and liver cancer.

Ms. Schuster worked as a machinist for Colfor, which produces hypoid driving shafts, transmission shafts and transfer case shafts. Her job entailed a lot of twisting and bending. One day at work she was changing the tools in a machine and twisted and turned. She felt something pop in her back. Ms. Schuster said, "I had instant pain down both legs and I couldn't hardly walk. I informed my foreman and he immediately took me to the office."

Her foreman filled out her paperwork and they asked her what she wanted to do. She said that she felt she had to go to the hospital because the pain was so intense.

Unable to walk, Ms. Schuster was put on a cart and driven to her car, but she had to drive herself. No one from the company helped or went with her. In severe pain, she did not think she could make it to the hospital and headed straight home. Ms. Schuster barely made it, and struggled to get into the front door. She asked her ailing husband, Sidney, to drive her to the hospital.

Ms. Schuster was examined at the hospital and X-Rays were ordered, but did not reveal anything serious. An MRI was not ordered at this time. The doctor prescribed a muscle relaxer, a painkiller and told her that she had suffered a strain in her back. She was sent home and referred her to AultWorks.

Here is a glimpse of the American health care future. As in Ms. Schuster's case, let us look at how the system really operates and is the role model for the United States. Colfor contracts with AultWorks to send their injured workers to their Urgent Care facility. Then their doctors and the doctors at Omni Orthopedics see the injured workers. Those doctors are on staff at Aultman Hospital, where the orthopedic surgeries are performed and where the injured workers have to receive physical therapy and rehabilitation. It is easy to see the foundation for enormous kickbacks. There is also a price to pay if the injured worker is dissatisfied with any of the AultWorks doctors. If they leave, according to Dr. Nichols and evidenced by reports gathered by this investigation, the Medical Director for Aultcomp, Dr. Michael Marvin, writes a terse file review which allegedly states that the injured worker does not need any more treatment, even if that is not the case.

Dr. Nichols stated, "Remember, the goal is to drive up the cost of care as quickly as possible without the employer realizing what is about to hit them in their premium rate spiking!

"Physical therapy costs $200 per hour. Most injured workers begin with one hour of PT that progresses to four hours of PT unsupervised, which costs $800 per day times 3 days a week at $2400 a week. Now times that by 20 people/day and you have $48,000 per day for AultWorks." Those figures add up to $192,000 per month that goes directly to AultWorks. Therefore, if an employer like Colfor fills AultWorks coffers, the doctors there are beholding to the company and normally find in the employer's favor and hang the injured worker out to dry. The evidence trail in Ms. Schuster's case makes that apparent.

Ms. Schuster was off three nights. Once seen at AultWorks, she was put on limited duty. Due to her husband's medical needs, Ms. Schuster had to keep working, but she tried to get her benefits.

That was not an easy task and she needed to get an attorney to help her through the process. Colfor was fighting the claim insisting the injury did not happen at work. Ms. Schuster hired Tracey Laslo, an Alliance, Ohio lawyer, but she never really saw her. Ms. Schuster's case was passed off to an assistant, Jim Black, who was not an attorney, but supposedly handled workers' compensation cases.

In order for her case to go forward, Ms. Schuster had to supply her medical records to the Laslo firm. They requested the records, which were needed because of a hearing that was scheduled for her claim. AultWorks would not release the records to them. Ms. Schuster called AultWorks and asked them to have the files ready because she wanted to pick them up, but when she arrived, AultWorks refused to give the records to her. Due to the kickback platform AultWorks had in place with Colfor, it is easier to understand their reluctance to help Ms. Schuster.

Without the medical records, Ms. Schuster could not prove that her injuries were work related despite the fact that she never had back injuries prior to her employment with Colfor. Black went to the hearing without the records and the case was dismissed immediately.

When Black told Ms. Schuster the case was dismissed, she was concerned that her claim was never going to be reopened. Although Black said that was not the case, they were still at the beginning of a very long fight and Mr. Schuster's fight was nearing its climax.

Ms. Schuster had a challenging juggling act in trying to care for her husband, to keep a job and to find relief for her increasing pain. She found another doctor, Dr. Lavender, who examined her and found that her injury was work related. He wanted an MRI to be done in order discover the root of her pain.

Colfor would not approve of the MRI. Without their approval, Ms. Schuster had little choice, but to resume work. "Working was pure pain," she told Dr. Nichols in a videotaped interview. She had to take pain pills to make it through her shift. Colfor did not care that she had to use a narcotic and work around dangerous equipment, which placed her and her coworkers in danger. Colfor also knew of Mr. Schuster's serious health issues, yet they did nothing to help Ms. Schuster. The shifts at Colfor were twelve hours long and she had to push herself. At times, she was forced to lean into tables just to stand up because her legs could no longer hold her. She told Dr. Nichols that she prayed for morning to come, the end of her shift. By the time she left the plant, she could hardly walk.

When she arrived home it added more stress for Mr. Schuster to see his wife in such a horrible condition and in excruciating pain. Still, Colfor did not budge in helping her. Her attorney was not much better. Ms. Schuster placed over 75 calls to the firm trying to get help, and none of her calls were returned. To get an answer about her case, she had to go in person and finally was told that the firm had not even filed an appeal in her case, delaying her treatments even further. She then went to see Mark Heinzerling, Jonathan Goodman's partner.

During the battle, it was discovered that Mr. Schuster was suffering from liver cancer and only had six months to live. Ms. Schuster needed to be home for her husband, but she also needed to work. Her back, however, got worse. To complicate the issue, Colfor repeatedly lost her paperwork or claimed that they did not have her paperwork, still insisting that her injury was not work related. On one occasion, a Colfor employee who was handling her claim denied ever having seen an accident report for Ms. Schuster, although she read straight from the report when talking to Ms. Schuster.

Finally, Ms. Schuster got an MRI, which confirmed that she had two fractures in her back. Now the fight began for her to get the surgery she needed, which was a laminectomy and fusion. That was a tremendous battle, but the battle at home was getting worse.

It was during this time that Dr. Nichols' compelling interview with Ms. Schuster was made. She sat next to her husband and as she spoke about the legal battle to get treatments, she kept her hand on her husband. Mr. Schuster was hooked up to oxygen and although he was having a difficult day, struggled to get his feelings across to Dr. Nichols about the maltreatment his wife had received from Colfor. He did not think about himself, only about her. For the most of the moving interview, Ms. Schuster remained tethered by love to her husband of 34 years. She was more worried about caring for him than for her own condition and being able to pay for his medication when she was not able to work. Ms. Schuster spoke about the difficulties of trying to care for him with her injured back and the torture of trying to get out of her chair at a moment's notice to help him. The couple's frustration was as palpable as their love for one another.

In the week following the interview, Mr. Schuster's condition rapidly declined. Caught in a whirlwind of emotions and pain, Ms. Schuster did all she could for him, but she could see her husband did not want to let go. He told her that he was worried that she would not get the help she needed and he did not want to leave her. He told her, "I just want you to be treated like a human being."

One day Ms. Schuster went to her husband's bedside, held his hand and told him that it was all right if he wanted to let go, that she would be fine. A little over an hour later, Mr. Schuster died breaking the tether.

Thrown into indescribable grief, agonizing pain, and feeling terribly alone, Ms. Schuster was lost. Colfor did nothing to help her, although her fellow employees took up a collection for her. Mr. Schuster did not have life insurance because of his condition, compounding her financial woes. Her health issues were very slow to be addressed. If it had not been for her regular insurance, Ms. Schuster would not have been able to get any assistance because Colfor made it impossible to get any benefits.

Ultimately, Ms. Schuster did receive back surgery, which offered her some help. Her finances never did recover and she had to file bankruptcy. In order to support herself, Ms. Schuster had to go back to work at Colfor. When you live in a small town, the options are minimal for other employment opportunities.

She did manage to get another position at Colfor, but it was no less demanding physically and she is now faced with surgery for severe carpal tunnel in both hands as a result of her work. Her doctors, including Dr. Nichols, have told her that she needs to quit her job before it kills her. With few openings in the job market, Ms. Schuster is left searching for alternatives to an impossible situation. The only benefit she received from Colfor and the BWC was $500 for her back. If it were not for her insurance, things would be a lot worse.

Still she feels suicidal and battles feelings of hopelessness. Doctors have her in pain management, but it is a vicious circle that could easily result in more serious problems.

Well aware of where she is emotionally right now, Dr. Nichols and his wife take her out to lunch and check on her, but she is in a precarious position, not unlike hundreds of thousands of people across the country.

Unfortunately, this method of treating the sick and injured workers of America is part of a larger plan that will change the face of the world in the next few years. There are corporations and foundations throughout the world that have a vested interest in weakening the work force and in many cases deliberately causing the deaths of multitudes around the world.

There is a reason that many of the injured workers feel suicidal and the reasons go well beyond the psychological sequelae of their injuries. It is time to look at the fact that many of these people have been brought to the brink of suicide intentionally. It also time to investigate the reason that the injured workers that receive the worst care are often vets and organ donors, like the injured workers already mentioned. It is time to investigate the people and the groups that are behind this plan. Is it possible that injured workers, sick and disabled Americans are guinea pigs viewed as less than human because of something more sinister, something so horrific that it will make the Holocaust seem small in comparison? The following chapters will help you to decide.

CHAPTER NINE
TOTAL CONTROL

There are powerful forces wielding their influence not only on the BWC in Ohio, but also on doctors and patients in this country and also around the world. Those forces have been working towards a goal for the past sixty years. They have morphed into several different entities in hopes of masking their affiliations and their intent, which is to take total control. Of course, on a smaller scale such as in national health care and in the various aspects of it like Workers' Compensation, they already have a large degree of control. However, that is not enough for these powerbrokers who will not stop until their command is absolute.

Forceful groups that are closely associated with these entities are the pharmaceutical companies, both American and European, which now comprise the largest lobbying group in Washington and have been exerting extreme pressure on Congress during the health care debate. These Big Pharma groups are not only working for their bests interests, but are also carrying out a carefully constructed manifesto that should concern every individual in this country.

In the previous chapters, it has been demonstrated that injured workers develop depression and anxiety partially related to their injuries and the frustration of the financial problems that result. Invariably, the injured worker is given antidepressants and tranquilizers in due haste without discussing the problems or giving them a chance to work through them. Due to countless delays and appeals, injured workers do not get the care they need and end up trying to get help for the overwhelming depression by seeing their Physician of

Record. The physician can then recommend psychological testing or prescribe antidepressants in the attempt to change the emotional outlook of the patient. Injured workers receive these medications much faster than they do treatment for their actual injuries. Once on these medications, the workers' compensation claims change from the physical injury to a psychological problem that helps the BWC keep its costs down and keeps the injured worker from ever getting the necessary treatments. These claims are not normally approved because they are considered Non-Allowable conditions, conditions that would not be present if treatment had been expedited.

Doctors use the DSM-IV, the Diagnostic and Statistical Manual of Mental Diseases to establish a so-called diagnosis, so the doctor can get paid and justify writing the script. That diagnosis labels the injured worker as depressed, psychotic or suicidal, even though the condition or state might only be temporary or merely a glimpse of something similar to exasperation over their circumstances. Like Diane Ferro who voiced her frustration about the lack of care to an IME doctor and found herself at a hospital for psychiatric evaluation only to have the examiner find she was not really suicidal at all, similar moments of frustration expressed by injured workers can be misinterpreted. Once that happens, they are smacked on prescription drugs that make the possibility of suicide all the greater and the risk of death even higher.

There might be a reason that the doctors readily hand out prescriptions for psychotropic drugs as if they were candy. With regard to injured workers, some doctors believe the medications will make life more tolerable during the grueling claims process, but as a whole, there are other factors at play. These factors are particularly found in cases throughout the population.

In interpreting the intricacies of a choreographed dance the doctors perform, we must look at their dance partners, the pharmaceutical companies, the powers behind them and their true intentions. A close relationship also exists between these pharmaceutical companies, the BWC and insurance companies throughout the world.

Historically, changes have been made over the past forty years that reflect a modification in how some specialties of medicine are practiced globally and specifically in developed countries. There has been a critical shift away from or a complete rejection of the Hippocratic Oath, as evidenced in part by the case studies already mentioned. While not all doctors subscribe to this modern technique, any doctor that writes a prescription without proper research into the drug being prescribed is an unwitting underwriter of this new methodology, a methodology designed to kill. Any doctor receiving kickbacks from pharmaceutical companies for writing prescriptions that are harmful to their patients is a full partner in the conspiracy.

Fifty years ago, life altering events such as illness, injury, death, divorce or financial problems were normally worked through and discussed with family, friends and sometimes a member of the clergy. Pills were not prescribed for situations that normally occur in one's life. All that changed in the 1960's. In 1967, a foundation was laid that has had a devastating impact on the population. A group of psychiatrists met in Puerto Rico to discuss how they could change their profession and bring it out of the basement of modern medicine and put it into the corner office and give it a position of real power. Working in conjunction with some influential organizations, this group of doctors crossed the line of ethics and in essence made a diabolical deal that would control large segments of the population and would have the potential to eliminate them.

At that meeting, Dr. Wayne O. Evans said, "We are developing potential for nearly a total control of human emotional states, mental functioning and will to act." If we think this meeting is something that should be relegated to the Twilight Zone, we need to think again. The main goal of this group and their platform was clear and concise. These psychiatrists, with the backing of their sponsors, wanted to be able to manipulate and to police every aspect of human behavior by the year 2000. We cannot discount what Evans said. In the 1960's, he was the Director of the Military Stress Laboratory in Natick, Massachusetts. He and his colleagues were part of a study group examining the Effects of Psychotropic Drugs on Normal Humans, and the group sponsored the meeting in Puerto Rico.

Evans went on to say, "If we accept that human mood, motivation, and emotion are reflections of a neuro-chemical state of the brain, then drugs can provide a simple, rapid expedient means to produce any desired neuro-chemical state that we wish." Dr. Evans ideas only expanded upon the beliefs held by psychiatrists in the early 20th Century. "Social Planners" during that time firmly believed that mind-altering drugs would be used to control the population.

Bertrand Russell considered one of the founding fathers of analytic philosophy and a social theorist said, "Diet, injections and injunctions will continue from a very early age to produce the sort of character and the sort of beliefs that the authorities consider desirable. And any serious criticism of the powers that be will become psychologically impossible."[58]

The CIA agreed with Russell in many ways and had been interested for some time with the effects of LSD on the population and experimented quite freely since 1947. Working on drug experiments that were intended to subvert the cultures of other countries not in alliance with the United States, the CIA and their adjunct psychiatrists were also busy subverting the American culture as well. Experiments were conducted on both military and civilians.

Surprisingly, independent psychiatrists were also interested in how drugs could manipulate the human mind and one of the most profound test cases involved two doctors at the Haight-Ashbury Clinic in San Francisco during the 1960's. Dr. Roger Smith and Dr. David E. Smith, who were not related, decided

---

[58] The Impact of Science on Society by Sir Bertrand Russell

to take drug testing a step further and instead of using rats, made the choice to test humans and their reactions to various drugs. One of their guinea pigs arrived at the clinic right out of prison. His name was Charles Manson and Roger Smith was his parole officer. Before Manson came along, the two doctors were carrying out experiments on rats forced to live in crowded conditions. They studied the violence the rats exhibited and then administered amphetamines to the rats to see how that would change the dynamics of rats in their confined space. The rats on the drugs quickly became killers and took out large segments of the rat population.

With Manson, the doctors had nearly the perfect test subject. He had come from a broken home and had been in prison much of his life. Manson was already looking for ways to control people to carry out his criminal intentions. Having studied mind control, hypnosis and manipulation, he was actively seeking a way to put a group together that would become his "family." Of course we know how his story turned out, but what we might not know is that some of the material used by Manson to create a deadly killing machine was also the guiding force behind the Evans group and the CIA projects.

Using concepts straight from Aldous Huxley's Brave New World and incorporating some of H.G. Wells' concepts, Manson took killing to a new level, but the vehicle that got the family into the mindset Manson desired was drugs.

Dr. Evans statements about controlling the total behavior of humans by 2000 also were reminiscent of Huxley and Wells. Evidence suggests that we have entered a new and dangerous phase in this country brought about by the willful manipulation of the population. Back in 1967, Evans' statements might have seemed preposterous. Today his assertions do not seem so farfetched. In Texas for instance, 66 percent of children in the foster care system were placed on psychotropic cocktails supposedly diagnosed as "very, very sick," by Joe Burkett MD, the head of the Texas Society of Psychiatric Physicians. Testifying before the Senate in Texas, he explained why the children were supposedly sick. He said, "They came from bad gene pools." He claimed that the children were in the foster care system because their parents were not responsible people, and for that reason the children were judged to be "sick" and were forced to take medication they did not need.[59] This incident in Texas is only a small part of what is happening globally and will be discussed in more depth, but it is a good indication that the psychiatrists' plans were well in place and that their goals were met.

If we look at the fact that psychotropic drugs help pharmaceutical companies rake in nearly a trillion dollars per year, we can assume the

---

[59] Houston Chronicle, October 27, 2004, Groups Criticize Remark about 'Bad Gene Pools' Doctor says his Statement about foster children not meant to offend, by Polly Ross Hughes

psychiatrists with the help of Big Pharma are well on their way to achieving their goal. According to estimates by IMS Health, drug sales in 2009 could reach $750 billion in a perniciously anemic economy.

How did they do it?

First, it must be understood that psychiatry is not based on real science. It is a specialty formed by observing behaviors of patients, analyzing and comparing that to established behaviors. The end result of those observations is supposedly a bona fide diagnosis, when in actuality it is an educated guess. Rarely do psychiatrists look for physical ailments present in the patient that could bring about emotional or mental problems. There are no blood tests or other testing mechanisms that can prove a patient is suffering from one mental disorder or another. Any diagnostic tests that are administered have come under fire even by psychiatrists because they are not necessarily precise assessments of the patients. Normally, a psychiatrist does not spend much time with a patient and as a whole; the visit is limited to no more than a few minutes. Therefore, their assessment cannot have any scientific basis, but instead only a subjective one. Consequently, those evaluations could be highly inaccurate. In an unspoken maxim from that meeting in 1967, accuracy was not as important as dependency. In essence, the framework of the psychiatrists' plan was to ensure dependency, which would be a permanent partner. That dependency would ensure an ever growing patient base for themselves and lifetime customers for the pharmaceutical companies. The problem was how would they be able to control the minds of the population by the year 2000 when at the time, psychiatry was on the periphery of medicine.

The answer was simple. Create more disorders. Note the term create rather than discover new disorders. How would these psychiatrists revolutionize their field and create disorders?

Psychiatrists would get together and by consensus develop a laundry list of disorders, ones that might not be abnormalities at all, but rather normal human behavior that they would christen as a psychological disturbance that should be treated. Of course, that treatment would consist of psychotropic drugs. The pharmaceutical companies were asked to dance and they gladly put on their tap shoes and created medications for the alleged disorders.

To see how their plans progressed, we can compare the DSM-IV Manual that was created in 1952 to today's manual to see just how the psychiatrists have used their imagination to our detriment.

In 1952, the DSM was put together by agreement following a vote. It was about 130 pages long and listed 106 disorders. Today the DSM-IV Manual has 934 pages and lists nearly 400 disorders, but the number is growing continually. The changes in the number of psychotropic drugs also increased from 44 in 1966 to more than three times that amount today. The end is not even in sight for new disorders and new medications because drug companies want to keep the cash flowing freely into their companies. So psychiatrists will convene again and decide on new disorders for which new drugs will have to be developed or at least old drugs will be renamed, given a new color and new promotion as the latest and greatest advance towards fighting a spurious disease.

Although drug companies claim that they must spend enormous amounts of money on research and development, actual figures dispute those claims. In some cases, drug companies spend as little as 11% of their revenues on R & D. The pharmaceutical company, Merck, had profits that were three times the amount spent for research and development.[60] All we have to do is to look at the employment numbers for R & D and compare them with those of marketing and it is clear where the drug companies' priorities lie. In 2000, American drug companies employed 48,527 in R & D, but in marketing, the companies employed 87,810.[61]

There are very few new drugs that are developed and as patents run out for the pharmaceutical blockbusters like Paxil, Zoloft and other mega-selling drugs, the pharmaceutical companies are desperate to perpetuate the illusion about innovation and scientific discovery, desperate to keep the money machine operating at full capacity. Expected patent expirations for 2011 and 2012 are estimated to be quite large and thus will necessitate a scramble by pharmaceutical companies to find something new or recycled. Interesting to note that from 1989 to 2000, 65 percent of new drugs that the FDA approved contained the same compounds as medications already on the market.[62] Further, the prices of drugs have increased in double digit percentages and will likely increase even more in the coming years, but this is not because more money is needed for research and development, but rather it is a question of greed. To guarantee the drug companies stay in the black, consumers are hit hard by their hard-selling approach used in marketing their drugs.

Consumers are targeted about the virtually countless psychological disorders through huge advertising campaigns that tell us we are sick. Television commercials highlight normal feelings that everyone has experienced during our lives. For instance, we sit in front of the television and hear the question directed toward us, "Are you afraid to speak in front of a lot of people?" Or this question, "Do you get nervous in new situations?" The answers to both questions of course would be yes. We all feel that way on occasion. Immediately, we get the diagnosis that we have Social Anxiety Disorder, and if that is too specific, then we might have General Anxiety Disorder. There is supposed hope though because we are told there is help for

---

[60] Profiting from Pain: Where Prescription Drug Dollars Go, A report by Families USA 2002

[61] Drug Industry Marketing Staff Soars While Research Staffing Stagnates, by Alan Sanger and Deborah Socolar, December 6, 2001 Boston: Health Reform Program, Boston University School of Public Health

[62] Profiting from Pain: Where Prescription Drug Dollars Go, A rep ort by Families USA 2002

this fictitious mental disorder and we start to buy into it. Without challenging the information we are force-fed, we accept the fact that we are ill and need medication in spite of the fact we are experiencing normal emotions and feelings. We are being told those emotions and feelings are abnormal by the psychiatric community and the pharmaceutical companies. Without reservation, we believe the marketing ploy and hurry to make an appointment with our doctor so that we can carry out the mantra, "Ask your doctor about whether our drug is right for you." Although this question has seen fantastic results, a different approach was launched recently by AstraZeneca Pharmaceuticals that is sure to reap huge profits. Their foreboding slogan, "Bipolar Depression can consume you," is bound to panic people and send them in droves to their doctors to ask for Seroquel XR. We will see even more disturbing advertising gimmicks in the near future all carefully thought out to achieve the highest monetary return. To perfect their plans and to facilitate their marketing campaigns, Big Pharma would not be content with just psychiatrists peddling their pills.

They launched personal campaigns targeting all physicians that meet with drug representatives. Those representatives always arrive bearing gifts and promises of remuneration for the prescriptions written for their products. Sadly, most doctors comply with their requests and acquiesce when we tell the doctor we are suffering from one or more fictitious disorders. Since we cannot be tested to determine the accuracy of our assumptions, the physician normally goes along with our requests. Over 70% of all psychotropic drugs are prescribed by general practitioners.

The total number of people worldwide on psychotropic medication is estimated at over 100 million people. To put that into perspective, that is nearly 33 percent of the American population. Big Pharma will do what it takes to keep those dollars rolling in and keeping any bad press or concerns about side effects to a minimum. Therefore, people will take these dangerous drugs without realizing the serious repercussions that go with them. Psychiatrists and general practitioners should know about them. It is a safe bet that the drug companies know that these drugs are deadly. Some chemists that worked in the industry have attested to the fact that the many of these drugs are not safe for human consumption and are actually lethal.

Nevertheless, the medical community has been deceived into thinking the pills are safe because of reports published in major medical journals, which claim the drugs are completely safe, if taken as prescribed, but they do not tell doctors that the authors of those papers and studies are on the pharmaceutical payroll. When it comes to responsibly informing patients of the harmful side effects and the possibility of death, the medical community has been terribly remiss.

Parents have seen their children deteriorate when taking anti-depressants and Attention Deficit Disorder medication to the point that the children's behavior becomes almost unrecognizable. Some of the children have committed suicide while taking the medication. Asked about whether they knew the drugs could kill or lead to suicide, most parents said they had no idea that could happen. Very few parents or patients are informed that the drugs can lead to homicide as well, let alone the serious diseases that can result after taking these psychotropic drugs. No one in their right mind would willingly take a drug with such dangerous side effects and that is why the pharmaceutical companies spend billions in advertising or brainwashing designed to focus on the utopian aspects of treatment. They emphasize how happy people are when taking their particular drug. Side effects are unimportant to drug companies. They only want lifetime customers. Since these bogus diseases have no cure, they can only be "managed." Therefore, the drug companies have practically guaranteed their longevity.

Unfortunately, small children are being targeted as well, often without parental knowledge. New tests have been developed that are horribly skewed and are certainly not scientifically based. These tests are administered allegedly to determine whether or not our children are depressed, suicidal or have Attention Deficit Disorder. One such test developed by Dr. David Shaffer was so skewed that 84% of the children taking the test were deemed suicidal. Even by Shaffer's own admission, the test was inaccurate. It should come as no surprise that Shaffer has ties to major pharmaceutical companies.

Other tests are now being used in 500 American cities and in 43 states. It does not stop there. Drug testing on children has become common place and consequently we are hearing about bipolar disease in young children, although most ethical doctors agree that children do not have bipolar disease. Yet, with enough advertising, and there are reports that drug companies spend over $5 billion per year on ad campaigns, the public is conditioned to buy into the lies without question and as a result, children are needlessly placed on medication.

When children are diagnosed with Attention Deficit Disorder or ADD, they are not told that nutrition plays a major role in their child's behavior. They are not told that blood tests can determine the cause of the symptoms associated with short attention spans. Often by removing gluten from a child's diet or limiting the amount of sugar a child consumes attention spans lengthen and symptoms are alleviated or eliminated, but that is not what drug companies want for our children. Instead, doctors hand out prescriptions that could kill and at the very least have very disturbing side effects, especially in children.

Injured workers have fallen into the medication pit because doctors perceive that it is the best way to treat ensuing depressions following injuries, instead of pushing the BWC and MCO's to allow surgery or proper treatments. The injured workers are placed on high-powered psychotropic medications to help with depression and pain, and in a sense, it silences the injured worker by inducing a medicated stupor that leads the worker into a dark and distressing future devoid of hope. The real answer would be to allow the surgery; the treatments and the physical therapy that would lead the injured worker back to work. With the way the system works now that is out of the question and there are some distressing reasons for this chosen course.

Injured workers, just like millions of Americans, are being given dangerous drugs that are not properly tested. We assume these drugs are deemed safe otherwise they would not be prescribed. However, that is not the case.

The Food and Drug Administration or the FDA is responsible for testing medications in this country. The FDA's panel of experts decides which medications will be approved and that should only be done after proper testing and hopefully then reach an unbiased decision. That is not possible at the FDA today because the members of the panel are known to have close associations with pharmaceutical companies making any scientific and fair evaluation unlikely. Many of these doctors receive money either in grants for research or outright salaries from drug companies for promoting and lecturing about their products. Consequently, there is a major conflict of interest present at the outset of any drug testing taking place in the United States today.

It used to take years for drugs to get FDA approval. Now it is less than two years and in many instances that time has been cut to a few short months, hardly enough time to determine toxicity or long-term effects the drugs might have on consumers. It is all about money. In the past, an application for a new drug registered with the FDA for approval had a fee of $100,000. Today, a new drug application commands a $1 million fee. We can see where this leads. With all the purported new drugs out there that are sent to the FDA for approval, it is easy to see the FDA is doing quite well.

To date, we are hit by an advertising barrage to get us to take psychotropic drugs. Still, there is a time that is quickly approaching, thanks to new legislation, which will mandate psychological testing for all Americans. There is also a new bill that has passed the House of Representatives and is now in the Senate under S. 324. If this bill becomes law, women giving birth will be tested for mental illness before they are allowed to take their babies home. While the current piece of legislation indicates new mothers can opt out, there is a door left open for the possibility that the testing of the mother will become mandatory and will be ongoing throughout the child's life. This bill is in response to the problems that some women face and psychiatry has coined as Post-Partum Depression. It is even possible, given certain test findings that the baby would not be allowed to leave the hospital with the mother. We can almost be assured that mandatory drug treatment will be ordered.

Are drugs making things worse for injured workers? Dr. Nichols has seen his patients go down a treacherous trail from heavy-duty narcotics to the psychotropic drugs that are prescribed to deal with the depression and anxiety. Once the patients start on those drugs supposedly to treat the depression and anxiety they are experiencing, there is deterioration in their mental and emotional state. An injured worker that struggles with the life altering events of an injury and being out of work can develop suicidal thoughts because the BWC process is so convoluted and stacked against them. Adding psychotropic medication can compound those feelings of suicide and worthlessness putting the injured worker at even greater risk for suicide. At the very least, as seen with the Bill Durst case, the medication is just too much for the heart to take.

Psychotropic drugs should not be taken long-term, but doctors have a tendency to overlook that point. If an injured worker wants to get off the psychotropic medication that could involve hospitalization because there are terribly risky side effects such as convulsions that can result from a rapid removal of the medication. One of Dr. Nichols' patients had his psychotropic medications cutoff arbitrarily without providing him a hospital setting for withdrawal, which placed the man at tremendous risk.

By denying treatments and battling the injured worker over the course of several years, the injured worker is placed into a gloomy emotional corner. Evidence shows that the BWC and the MCOs are well aware of the risks for heart attack; liver failure and suicide risks are much higher when psychotropic medications are prescribed. The unwillingness to treat injured workers in a timely manner compels many of these people to find something they believe will help them handle their problems. Again, heavy pharmaceutical advertising on television seems to guarantee the injured workers can beat their depression and feel better about themselves and be happy.

If we look at the figures for injured workers throughout this country, we can get a better idea just how much of a problem there could be with psychotropic and pain medication. In 2000, 26 million American workers went to see their doctors for back problems, 7 million of those workers suffered from low back pain. Those workers seeking medical help for knee pain numbered 17 million the same year. Shoulder problems accounted for 12 million workers who visited physicians and 13 million workers sought help for foot and ankle problems. An estimated 3.4 million people filled doctors' offices complaining of carpal tunnel syndrome.[63] It would be safe to say that the majority of these American workers were given one or more medications for their injuries. Therefore, there is a great deal of profit to be made for pharmaceutical companies.

Injuries, whether they happen on the job or not can adversely affect a person's lifestyle. Yet, the way the BWC, the MCOs and employers care for the injured worker is directly related to the length of time the treatment takes and consequently how long it takes for depression and/or suicidal thoughts to develop. According to the Employer Manual, it states, "Negative thought increases sympathetic response, which decreases the injured worker's immune system. In a sense, if the immune system is compromised, the worker is injury

---

[63] National Center for Health Statistics, National Ambulatory Care Survey, 2000

prone or may already have an injury and require prolonged care. Thus this works both ways. Positive thought and input from the employer and treating doctor will generally improve the injured worker's recovery rate and facilitate early return-to-work simply by boosting the worker's immune response to the trauma."[64] Nevertheless, the practice of the BWC, MCOs, physicians and psychiatrists is to medicate.

The cradle to tomb approach to mental health and health care in general is the well-conceived brainchild of Big Pharma, many psychiatrists, insurance companies and the government as well. Their acquired attitude is to view the injured or the sick as an expendable commodity. Viewed as weak and in need of "care," patients are ushered into a clinical serfdom of sorts and placed into a position of having to rely on the overlords of medicine to help them. A Gallup poll in June 2009 showed that 73 percent of Americans believe that they can trust their doctors. The poll results offer convincing proof that the majority of us could swallow whatever we are told even if it is not in our best interests. We readily turn the reins over to someone who might not be worthy of our trust. An unethical practioner's first choice of action is to keep a patient in a sort of cocoon and to liberally medicate the person. Most people readily accept the medications unaware of specific plans put in place by the pharmaceutical companies and by some people within the medical community.

Statistics show that patients that have been diagnosed with Major Depression were frequent users of the health care system and their total medical costs, which include medical, disability and pharmaceutical costs were 4.2 times the amount for those not diagnosed with depression. Obviously pharmaceutical companies benefit from those people diagnosed with major depression and as such have a gold mine, if they can maintain their clients on psychotropic drugs.

The silent partner in this transformation has been the government, but that position will soon dissolve into a much more active and overt role. All of these partners count on our ignorance and our blind trust in modern medicine.

The World Health Organization estimated that by 2020, Mental Depression would come in a close second to cardiovascular disease. Think of the opportunities for the global pharmaceutical market if those estimates are correct. A question must be raised about whether this is actual mental depression or the results of skewed testing and mega-marketing on the part of pharmaceutical companies? The chances are quite good that governments will play a pivotal part in determining who is depressed and as we have seen, a portion of this can be accomplished through legislation and mandatory testing. In any event, we can see clearly the ultimate destination.

Screenings by employers are already happening in this country and when combined with the assault of advertising, the drug companies will grow even

---

[64] Employer Handbook for On-the-Job Injuries 2006

larger, and with that growth become even stronger lobbyists of governments. The loser here is the average person whose mental and physical health will be determined by governments mesmerized by pharmaceutical companies.

An interesting point to note is that depression shortens life expectancy. If we assume that patients are given anti-depressants to supposedly counteract the depression, but the side effects make the person further depressed, is not the medical community practically giving these patients death sentences by freely prescribing psychotropic medication? The answer is simple. Yes, that is exactly what happens.

The BWC is aware of the side effects of anti-depressants and the causal relationship between injury, depression and shortened life expectancy. As in the Bill Durst case, it could be safely argued that he was given those medications knowing full well his treatment would not be approved and knowing how that medication would affect his body.

Pain management and the pain medication that is prescribed quickly for injured workers have significant drawbacks too, especially if treatment is delayed or denied repeatedly. Here are some side effects of the commonly prescribed pain medications.

Oxycontin-Constipation, dizziness, drowsiness, dry mouth, headache, itching, nausea, sweating, vomiting, weakness abdominal pain, abnormal dreams, abnormal thoughts, anxiety, chills, confusion, diarrhea, dizziness upon first standing up, excessively high spirits, fever, hiccups, indigestion, insomnia, loss of appetite, nervousness, rash, stomach pain, shortness of breath, twitching abnormal gait, accidental injury, agitation, amnesia, burping, chest pain, cough, decreased sexual drive, dehydration, **Depression**, difficulty swallowing, diminished muscle tone, diminished sensitivity, dry or inflamed skin, emotional instability, fainting, gas, generally ill feeling, hallucinations, hives, impotence, increased appetite, intestinal obstruction, lack of menstruation, loss of identity, migraine, neck pain, over-activity, pain, ringing in the ears, seizures, sore throat, speech disorder, stomach problems, stupor, swollen arms and legs, swollen face or mouth, swollen lymph nodes, taste changes, thirst, tingling, tremor, urinary problems, vertigo, vision changes, voice changes, vomiting.[65]

Darvocet-Drowsiness, dizziness, nausea, sedation, vomiting, abdominal pain, constipation, feelings of elation or **Depression**, hallucinations, headache, kidney problems, light-headedness, liver problems, minor visual disturbances, skin rashes, weakness, yellowed eyes and skin.[66]

---

[65] Employers Handbook 2006
[66] ibid

Vicodin-Dizziness, light-headedness, nausea, sedation, vomiting, allergic reactions, anxiety, blood disorders, constipation, decreased mental and physical capability, **Depression**, difficulty urinating, drowsiness, fear, hearing loss, itching, mental clouding, mood changes, restlessness, skin rash, slowed breathing, sluggishness.[67]

Flexoril-Dizziness, drowsiness, dry mouth, abnormal heartbeats, abnormal sensations, abnormal thoughts or dreams, aggressive behavior, agitation, anxiety, bloated feeling, blurred vision, confusion, constipation, convulsions, decreased appetite, **Depression**, diarrhea, difficulty falling or staying asleep, difficulty speaking, disorientation, double vision, excitement, fainting, fatigue, fluid retention, gas, hallucinations, headache, heartburn, hepatitis, hives, increased heart rate, indigestion, inflammation of the stomach, itching, lack of coordination, liver diseases, loss of sense of taste, low blood pressure, muscle twitching, nausea, nervousness, palpitations, paranoia, rash, ringing in the ears, severe allergic reaction, stomach and intestinal pain, sweating, swelling of the tongue or face, thirst, tingling in hands or feet, tremors, unpleasant taste in the mouth, urinating more or less than usual, vague feeling of bodily discomfort, vertigo, vomiting, weakness, yellow eyes and skin.[68]

Ibuprofen-Abdominal cramps or pain, abdominal discomfort, bloating and gas, constipation, diarrhea, dizziness, fluid retention and swelling, headache, heartburn, indigestion, itching, loss of appetite, nausea, nervousness, rash, ringing in ears, stomach pain, vomiting, abdominal bleeding, anemia, black stool, blood in urine, blurred vision, changes in heartbeat, chills, confusion, congestive heart failure, **Depression**, dry eyes and mouth, emotional volatility, fever, hair loss, hearing loss, hepatitis, high or low blood pressure, hives, inability to sleep, inflammation of nose, inflammation of the pancreas or stomach, kidney or liver failure, severe allergic reactions, shortness of breath, skin eruptions or peeling, sleepiness, stomach or upper intestinal ulcer, ulcer of gums, vision loss, vomiting blood, wheezing, yellow eyes and skin.[69]

Vicoprofen-Abdominal pain, anxiety, constipation, diarrhea, dizziness, drowsiness, dry mouth, gas, headache, indigestion, infection, insomnia, itching, loss of strength, nausea, nervousness, sweating, swelling, vomiting, confusion, dark tarry stool, difficulty breathing, fever, flu symptoms, frequent urination, hiccups, inflammation of the throat and nasal passages, loss of appetite, mouth ulcers, pain, ringing in the ears, skin tingling, stomach inflammation, tension, thinking abnormalities, thirst,

---

[67] Employers Handbook 2006
[68] ibid
[69] Employers Handbook 2006

throbbing heartbeat, abnormal dreams, agitation, allergic reaction, altered vision, asthma, bad taste, bronchitis, chalky stool, decreased sex drive, **Depression**, difficulty swallowing, dry eyes, elevated mood, hives, hoarseness, impotence, increased cough, inflamed sinuses, inflammation of the tongue or intestines, joint pain, low blood pressure, lung congestion, mood changes, muscle ache, pneumonia, rapid or irregular heartbeat, rash, shallow breathing, skin swelling, slurred speech, teeth clenching, tremor, urinary problems, vertigo, weight loss.[70]

Percocet-Dizziness, light-headedness, nausea, sedation, vomiting, constipation, **Depression**, exaggerated feeling of well-being, itchy skin, skin rash, slowed breathing.

These pain medications all have similar side effects and depression is listed in each of these medications. While it might be necessary to manage pain in the short-term, any long-term use pain medication has serious emotional and physical consequences. The BWC understands those consequences and so do the pharmaceutical companies that those pain medications can be an unguarded gateway to psychotropic drugs.

Doctors normally try to limit the amount and duration of narcotic intake, however, chronic pain can change the game plan, particularly if treatment is delayed or refused. Statistics show that not all doctors are experienced in prescribing controlled substances to injured workers. A recent study was done by The National Center on Addiction and Substance Abuse (CASA) at Columbia University that looked at how much experience and education a regular physician receives when it comes to prescribing pain medication in a pain management setting.

The study listed the findings of a survey done asking physicians if they had received any education in medical school in the prescribing controlled substances to injured workers. Of those surveyed, only 55.4 percent of the doctors had received any training. Within that group, only 57.6 percent had only a few hours of training or less. The percentage of those doctors that received more than a few hours of training was 34.8 percent. How many physicians took the entire course? The answer was none.

When these doctors were asked if they had completed a pain management course in medical school, only 47.5 percent had taken the course. Those that completed the entire course were 5.2 percent.

During residency, the survey results showed that 69.9 percent had received some training in prescribing controlled substances to injured workers and only 10.3 percent had actually finished the course. Those that

---

[70] ibid

took a pain management course during their residency totaled 61.7 percent, but only 9.6 percent had completed the course.

The survey of doctors already in practice was a little more hopeful. Doctors that had taken Continuing Education Courses in prescribing controlled substances to injured workers were 44.5 percent, with 26.4 percent completing the course. The number of doctors that took CME instruction on pain management was 59.3 percent, but only 30.6 percent had finished the course.

The statistics are not very reassuring to injured workers or anyone in need of a pain management program. The numbers also explain why there are so many problems that arise during the course of treatment that could have been avoided with proper education and with the proper mindset of the BWC and MCOs.

The problem with improper and uneducated pain management is that all too often opioids are prescribed to counteract the pain. The downside is that it is only the perception of pain that is managed and does not address the real problem or injury. Chances of further injury are higher when patients take opioids like those listed above and mask the pain, which gives a false sense of wellbeing to the injured worker or patient. There are dangers involved when injured workers return to work while using narcotics and operate or are around machinery. They pose a danger not only to themselves, but also to their co-workers because the medications slow response times and perceptions.

The very nature of how the BWC does business is the true indication that pain management is the most profitable means for the bureau to acquire the profits it is seeking. The MCOs also believe in this modality because it greatly improves their bottom line. In clinical studies it is evident that if a worker does not return to work within a year, the chances for the injured worker returning drop 25 percent.[71] After two years of disability, the chances are slim that an injured worker will get back to work. Depression is also a key factor that delays healing and thus compounds the problem. The bureau knows this and perhaps that is why injured workers are not treated promptly because it assures the pharmaceutical companies of even more clients. As mentioned above, pain management has depression as one of its major disadvantages.

Dr. Nichols understands all too well just how the operation works and that is why he has come under such intense scrutiny and pressure. If we

---

[71] Waddell G, Allan DB, and Newton M: Clinical evaluation of disability in back pain, in Frymoyer, J.W. The Adult Spine: Principles and Practice, Raven Press, New York, 1991.

look at the fact in the first five years an injured worker is in the system, they are the responsibility of the employer. After that time, the responsibility shifts to the BWC. For that reason, we see the bureau doing everything it can to push the worker, treated or not, out the door before the BWC has to pick up the full tab for the worker's care. This mechanism has resulted in cruel and inhumane treatment of injured workers and in the cases of injured workers like Bill Durst; it has a high mortality rate. For the BWC, it is not the treatment of injured workers that is vital, but rather it is the cost of claims, which must be driven up in order to sustain the bureau's investment goals and the political coffers. This can be evidenced in the bureau's large footprint found on Wall Street.

MCOs have assisted in driving up claims, which helps the BWC in its goals. The BWC and the MCOs have an unholy alliance with the pharmaceutical companies. Together they prefer that injured workers go through pain management, which costs three times that of alternative care such as chiropractic, which is three times more effective at treating musculoskeletal injuries. The alliance reaps millions of dollars by sending injured workers down this avenue, which further debilitates them. This endless cycle only benefits the alliance and underscores the lack of value placed on the injured worker's life.

File reviewers and IME doctors have a pertinent role in keeping costs high. Without these key players, the bureau and the MCOs would not have the lucrative returns that they now enjoy. Legislation that is in place allows the MCOs a percentage of the employer's premium rate. The system, as Dr. Nichols put it is, "gamed." He said, "It doesn't take a rocket scientist to figure out that if you are going to get a percentage of a product, which in this instance is derived from a combination of cost factors such as cost of treatment, litigation cost etc…it is in your best interest to drive up the cost of that product in order to maximize your profit margin."

For the unholy alliance to survive it is critical for it to remain intact and that means that any threats to it must be quashed quickly. We are witnessing a developing battle to shove chiropractic out of the picture. This movement is spearheaded by the pharmaceutical companies that will not tolerate alternative forms of healing or more precisely, any treatment that does not consist of drug therapy. There are attempts to drive the chiropractors out of the BWC system and several groups are trying to draft legislation to achieve that end in Ohio and in other parts of the country.

In Ohio, the BWC is taking this a step further in order to stop a decrease in injured workers. They are now trying to dismantle the Safety and Hygiene Division of the bureau because its main purpose is to prevent work injuries. Dr. Nichols stated, "This does not improve the Bureau's bottom line because less workers are becoming injured, which translates into less premium monies." According to a source within the Safety and Hygiene Division, the bureau has been allegedly embezzling from them for some time, undercutting their budget and thus keeping them from promoting safety in the workplace. Since the employees have raised concerns with Marsha Ryan, Director of the Bureau, the dismantling plans have been drawn up allegedly to cover up the embezzlement. Ryan was appointed by Governor Strickland and it is already been evidenced that the appointment is politically expedient. The pharmaceutical industry is a major campaign contributor and it has a vested interest in protecting its sacred territory.

Throughout the country we are seeing any encroachment on pharmaceutical territory having severe ramifications and we are also witnessing unprecedented moves by the pharmaceutical companies to thwart any treatments that do not include prescription drug therapy.

Yet, something much more insidious is behind a major transformation in health care that has largely remained in stealth mode. It has had its impact on how the BWC handles injured workers and how health care at large will be handled after December 31, 2009.

Major changes are on the way, but most people including members of Congress are unaware of what is going to happen here and around the world. The thunderclouds are gathering and the world is about to be engulfed in a storm of biblical proportions. We will lose our right to choose what we want or do not want to consume. This includes every bit of food we will eat, every nutritional supplement. Every food consumed by human or animal will be controlled, everything except pharmaceuticals.

As mentioned previously, certain groups have been working to establish control over various aspects of our lives, health care only being a small part of that. If we want to have an idea of what our future would be like, it is essential to discuss the plans of these groups and how they will impact our lives. We have seen a glimpse in how injured workers have been treated, but it is time to expand our view to see how even healthy people would be affected.

In 1962, five years prior to the fateful psychiatric meeting in Puerto Rico, decisions were made and steps taken to control everything the world population would consume. In marinating on the gravity of these landmark decisions, a brief history of the mastermind behind them is important.

In the years leading to World War II, work was already being in done in the chemical and pharmaceutical field in Germany that would lead to world domination and population control, not just as the Nazis envisioned it, but something on a much larger scale. IG Farben was a giant chemical and pharmaceutical company that was created after Bayer, BASF, Hoechst and other companies joined in a formidable corporation that would have a colossal impact on the world. IG Farben was instrumental in creating alternative fuel for the Nazis, which turned out highly farsighted after Germany's access to world oil supplies was severely limited during the war. The conglomerate also developed things like polyurethane and numerous kinds of drugs. They also made the steel for the Nazi railroad lines and the concentration camps.

Utilizing their chemical and pharmaceutical expertise, IG Farben created Zyklon B gas that was used in the extermination of the Jews. Fritz ter Meer worked for IG Farben and was on the executive committee. He was also on the technical committee and was the Director of Section II at Auschwitz during World War II. The camp must have suited ter Meer who was an avid believer in population reduction. In fact, one of IG Farben's plants was located in close proximity to Auschwitz.

During his term at the camp, women were sold to IG Farben at a price of 170 Reich Marks each so that pharmaceutical experiments could be conducted on them. The women were injected with supposed vaccines for Typhus and other diseases and the majority of them died. It is thought that the pharmaceutical monster experimented with many other drugs. IG Farben had also worked on fluoride projects before World War II and discovered that fluoride made people complacent. Many people would be shocked to learn that some of those experiments on fluoride led to its use in one of the major psychotropic drugs, Prozac, (fluoxetine hydrochloride) of which it is a key ingredient.[72] Many injured workers are prescribed Prozac for depression and it is known to have suicidal risks associated with it. Additionally, complacent injured workers do not complain or fight back effectively.

During the Nuremberg trials for crimes against humanity, ter Meer was found guilty of "enslavement" and "plundering" and was sentenced to seven years in prison. Prison did not change his obsession for controlling the population and in some ways his obsession grew stronger. After he was set free, ter Meer wasted no time in advancing his cause and the cause of many of his friends.

He approached some high powered friends with connections to the United Nations and discussed with them his belief on how the population could be controlled. It was ter Meer's premise that if you control the food in the world, you control the people. The United Nations was in complete agreement, as were the Rockefellers, who had a strong penchant for limiting

---

[72] www.drugs.com/pro/fluoxetine.html

the population and who helped develop eugenics[73] in the early 1930's. The Rockefellers and their foundations were in fact helping the Nazis with their sinister experiments several years prior to the outbreak of World War II. In 1932, the Rockefellers and their friends elected a Swiss psychiatrist, Ernst Rudin, the president of the Third International Conference on Eugenics and had worked for several branches of the Rockefeller foundations. They founded the Kaiser Wilhelm Institute for Anthropology, Eugenics and Human Heredity and Rudin was involved with that. He was commissioned by Hitler's Minister of the Interior to draft a sterilization law for Germany. Rudin and ter Meer were trained by the Rockefeller foundations to carry out cruel experiments involving different forms of population control, which were later utilized by the Nazis. The notion that the genocide was a German idea is not entirely accurate because it had its origins in the United States. The Rockefellers were instrumental in putting together the United Nations, which would adopt the foundation's population control platform. Ter Meer also played a significant role in convincing the UN about the myriad of options that could be used.

After having successfully established what ter Meer and the United Nations wanted to do with food, a new trade commission was formed in 1962 called Codex Alimentarius. That trade commission established over 4,000 guidelines pertaining to food, nutritional supplements, everything we ingest with the exception of pharmaceuticals. It was the aim of Codex to have global control of food by December 31, 2009, which at that time would make Codex guidelines mandatory.

The World Health Organization, or WHO, and the Food and Agricultural Organization or FAO, oversee, run and fund Codex Alimentarius at the behest of the United Nations. These organizations have been working hard to transition mere guidelines into mandatory laws. They got a great deal of assistance after the World Trade Organization was formed in 1994. The WTO wanted some way to decide trade disputes that arose and decided wholeheartedly on adopting Codex Alimentarius as its framework for those decisions. Now every member of the WTO must accept those mandatory guidelines. The WTO gives tremendous precedence to these codes and because of that disputes are settled in favor of those countries that adhere to Codex. Countries that do not embrace Codex lose the case regardless of any meritorious elements. This position has powerful economic effects on countries, which in turn makes the countries that are non-compliant rush to get adopt the Codex guidelines.

---

[73] Eugenics is the science of improving the human population by controlled breeding to increase the occurrence of desirable characteristics. Developed largely by Francis Galton as a method of improving the human race. Oxford Dictionary

Big Pharma, naturally, has had a lot to do with countries becoming compliant with Codex and has been part of this agenda along with the big chemical, medical and agricultural conglomerates since its inception.

There is legislation in this country that was passed in 1994 was an affront to the pharmaceutical industry and to the Congress that wanted to stop consumer access to dietary supplements and high potency vitamins, but Americans were outraged and the Congress did an about face. The Dietary Supplemental Health and Education Act of 1994 basically stated that American consumers could freely take and have access to all nutrients and herbs because they were classified as foods.

DSHEA was a major victory not only for consumers, but also for doctors who practice alternative medicine and believe that with the right nutritional supplements and enzymes, people could be healed. The battle lines were drawn as far as Big Pharma was concerned and consequently Codex suddenly declared nutritional supplements and minerals as poison or toxins in 1994. Therefore, people would have to be protected from them.

DSHEA should override that decision because it became law, but since 1994 there has been a legislative effort to get rid of the law so that the United States would be compliant with Codex immediately. On December 31, 2009 all the Codex guidelines will become mandatory worldwide leaving little choice for governments but to comply. Once again, Big Pharma and the groups behind population control will gain a very powerful upper hand. Nutrients, minerals and vitamins will become illegal, much like cocaine or heroin. Incidentally, fluoride will not be illegal.

The overall outcome of the December 31, 2009 deadline will be much more harmful to billions of people and the FDA has gone on the record stating that it will go along with the Codex implementation even if that means going against US law. All food must be irradiated unless it is obtained locally. Even organic food must be radiated. According to Codex, all dairy cows in the world must be given Monsanto's recombinant bovine growth hormone and that means that all the milk and butter in the world will be tainted with the hormone. Further, all animals in the world that are used for food must be given subclinical antibiotics and must be given exogenous growth hormones.

Pesticides in food previously outlawed can again be used and there will be nothing the FDA or other agencies can do to protect American consumers. The problem is also a critical one worldwide. As of 2001, 176 countries banned twelve deadly organic chemicals, nine of which are pesticides. Nevertheless, Codex has changed that and will now allow seven of the nine forbidden chemicals back into food. Any food containing these chemicals cannot be stopped at US borders because that would be a trade infraction against Codex and the WTO.

If a food crisis develops either through famine or war, nutritional foods cannot be shipped to help people in the affected areas. It will be illegal.

We will not have long to wait to see an impact on these changes. The WTO and the FAO in an epidemiology report estimate that these news laws will result in the deaths of three billion people. It is estimated that one billion people will die of starvation and two billion will die from preventable diseases brought about by poor nutrition.

Non-genetically modified food or non-GMO food will no longer be available, which is serious news for people worldwide that have severe allergic reactions to modified foods.

In the interim, pharmaceutical companies like Pfizer, Merck, GlaxoSmithKline, Wellcome and Bayer have purchased nutrient businesses worldwide in their effort to seize total control. As an important side note, Bayer makes sure that a wreath is laid over Fritz ter Meer's grave every All Saints Day, underscoring their approval of his master or final solution. His plan has come a long way since Auschwitz.

It was mentioned earlier about other groups that have an intense interest in helping the pharmaceutical companies to carry out their plans. One such entity is the Council on Foreign Relations started by JP Morgan, Paul Warburg and JD Rockefeller. The group is responsible for the takeover of the print and broadcasting media and is behind global population control. Its members can be found in all crucial positions of power like the White House, Congress and many corporations and like Big Pharma they want total control. The group feels quite strongly about achieving a major decrease in the population and they and their financiers like the Rockefellers have funded drug research that fosters sterilization through vaccinations and even embraced nuclear holocaust in order achieve their goal. The target is to decrease the number of people by 90 percent. Therefore it is not surprising to see that pharmaceutical companies that have been working for decades at controlling the population are corporate members of the Council on Foreign Relations.

Some of the Big Pharma companies that are corporate members of the Council on Foreign Relations are Pfizer, Merck and Company, Inc., GlaxoSmithKline and BASF, one of IG Farben's partners. Some CEO's of the pharmaceutical companies are also listed as individual members, like Charles A. Heimbold, Jr. who was the CEO of Bristol-Myers Squibb. In

2001, Mr. Heimbold made $74,890,918 and that did not include $76,095,611 of unexercised stock options.[74]

Heimbold has not been the only pharmaceutical executive hauling in big bucks during their years as chief executives, but he has been at the top of the list. In this time of economic crisis, it might be possible for people to understand exorbitant salaries if those companies were developing drugs that actually helped people or finding the cure for cancer or HIV. However, health does not pay, only disease pays. Further it is an even harder pill to swallow knowing that the drug companies are deliberately harming people and actively working to "hook" as many people as possible in the pursuit of Social Biology, which is today's more acceptable term for eugenics.

Recently, Dr. Nichols had been trying to get Lewis "Rex" Whan into a pain management program. He made a friendly bet with Rex that the drug treatment would be approved quickly. Without a problem, the treatment was approved immediately whereas Rex's other treatments have been repeatedly denied.

After exhaustive research, it became apparent that there was much more incentive for the BWC and MCOs to approve pain management for injured workers. The things that are happening within the bureau are reflective of the pharmaceutical companies' power and planning that is aimed at medicating the majority of the population. Research has also shown that greed on the part of the bureau has made it easy for them to sell out injured workers, to avoid treating them and to push them into inexorable drug therapy, but there is a surprising note that arose that augmented the relationship between the BWC and pharmaceutical companies.

The BWC had an opportunity to cash in on millions of dollars of pharmaceutical rebates, but did not take them until a report was released from the Office of the Ohio Inspector General. For some unknown reason, the BWC purchased millions dollars' worth of expensive drugs for injured workers over the past few years. During the period from July 2005 until September 2008, the bureau could have obtained a rebate of $14.5 million from drug manufacturers, which could have redeemed the bureau following its series of investment scandals.[75]

Inspector General Thomas Charles found out during his investigation that the BWC had discovered that it had paid for three very expensive medications that were used to treat injured workers for specific conditions

---

[74] http://www.allbusiness.com/company-activities-management/financial-performance/6356979-1.html
[75] Business First of Columbus, October 26, 2009 Report: Missed rebates, drug spending cost BWC millions by Matt Burns.

in 2006 that had not been cleared with the FDA. There was no word on whether the injured workers were seriously harmed by the medications. Supposedly an internal review done in 2007 uncovered some things that needed to be changed at the bureau. The investigation showed that the bureau could have made specific changes in pharmaceutical purchases that would have saved $5.5 million in 2008, but delayed implementing constraints for several months.

Charles' report also indicated that there were improprieties concerning a BWC pharmacy consultant who used his official email account for personal use. Personnel were added to the division that supposedly helped some severe management problems also found in the department.

In other problems regarding the management of the bureau's drug program, one of its top auditors thought that it was not clear if the $637 million that went through the BWC's prescription drug program were properly spent by ACS State Healthcare. ACS was the outside agency that the bureau hired to manage pharmacy benefits for Ohio's injured workers. The problem apparently arose around 2002. BWC funds were merged with 12 other ACS customer funds nationwide that left auditors concerned, especially when the auditors learned that ACS did not reconcile banking statements against the BWC's accounting records.[76]

In the 44 page audit report, ACS was given very poor marks in handling funds and failed to return over $300,000 in uncashed checks, did not monitor pharmacies on-site performance and did not collect rebates on drugs with no generic equivalent that could have saved $9 million annually. The bureau was also received some pointed comments regarding its failure to properly manage its funds and correctly oversee its operations.

Perhaps in an attempt to clean up its image, the BWC went a step further and made an interesting choice regarding pharmacy management when it signed a contract with SXC, a pharmaceutical management company, but there is more to this new partnership than just pharmaceutical management. This is a pertinent connection that Dr. Nichols also understands, but he is not alone.

A case involving Keith Ungar, DC, could attest to the fact that something is terribly wrong within the system and offer more proof of the corruption not only within the bureau, but also within the insurance and the pharmaceutical industries. Both industries promote their care and concern for their clients, but as we have seen, they take an adversarial role in dealing with them. Dr. Ungar, a far-sighted colleague of Dr. Nichols, has seen where all of the corruption is

---

[76] The Toledo Blade June 8, 2007 Audit reveals lax oversight for bureau of workers' comp

headed and has done his best to make it known that something is terribly wrong in this country.

He ran several chiropractic clinics throughout Ohio and was well-versed in how the bureau operated which was detrimental to his patients. Ungar assisted them, much like Dr. Nichols has done, when it came to IMEs and the bureaucratic baloney served freely by the bureau. Over the years, Dr. Ungar has gone into IME exams with his patients and served as a witness to the fraud committed by various IME doctors within the system. The doctors giving the examinations would assume he was a relative of the injured worker. Ungar would observe the exams and at times, would blow his cover when the doctor stepped out of bounds when the required testing was done inappropriately or not at all. He developed quite a reputation in the medical community as a maverick and at meetings; the corrupt doctors would never know when Dr. Ungar would call them out in the middle of a gathering accusing them of fraud and malfeasance.

Dr. Ungar could be considered a very pro-active injured worker advocate, someone who was feared by ethically challenged doctors. He never dreamed that one day he would be in a battle with the BWC, not as an advocate for an injured worker, but as an injured worker himself.

In January of 2005 he was treating a patient who weighed around 400 pounds. The patient began to fall off the treatment table and Dr. Ungar had to catch the patient. In doing so, he suffered a herniated disc in his lower back. Suddenly, he found himself in a dilemma shared by his patients. Hurt and unable to work, Dr. Ungar went through the process with the BWC as an employer and an injured worker.

Already knowing the belabored and unjust process of the bureau, Dr. Ungar knew what to expect, but he hoped that he could get help for his back. He had an MRI done, which clearly showed the disc had broken and dropped approximately 11 mm. He was in agony and his ordeal was not made any easier by his MCO.

Since 9/11, the BWC has access to motor vehicle records, perhaps a critical point in a complicated plan. In Dr. Ungar's case, the records were pulled and it was discovered that he had a slight fender bender in the parking lot of his office. One of his employees had backed out hitting his vehicle. No one was hurt and there was just minor damage done. However, the MCO made the case that Dr. Ungar had actually hurt his back at that time and not during the treatment of his patient as he claimed. It was a way of not only disputing the claim, but also accusing him of filing a false claim.

The case went to a hearing and was denied. Dr. Ungar was immersed in a monumental battle to save his practice and get help for his back. He felt that the MCO was denying a claim for a legitimate injury for financial gain. Unable to work on his patients as he had in the past, Dr. Ungar solicited the help of Dr. Nichols to help with treatments in his office. In misery, Dr. Ungar did all he could to alleviate the pain, but he was not about to take any medications for it.

All too aware of the dangerous side effects of drugs, Dr. Ungar did not take anything for his injury. He has spent his professional life learning and practicing natural medicine as a healthy alternative to the pharmaceutical racket, which made him a very large target of the BWC and the pharmaceutical companies. Like injured workers, his claim was fought down the line and when it came time to file for his disability insurance, he had another battle to fight, one that is still going on today. After several years of fighting, Dr. Ungar's credit rating was destroyed and he has experienced the unnecessary trials, frustrations and stress that other injured workers go through in their attempt for justice.

There has been an argument that the BWC has been able to intimidate some injured workers because of their lack of education, but Dr. Ungar's case proves that there is no class distinction and that even with all the necessary tools that Dr. Ungar has accumulated over the past twenty years in dealing with the BWC, they were not enough to stop the bureau of the MCO from thwarting him.

During the investigation of injured workers and their claims, it became apparent that there was a similarity in how some injured workers were treated quite well and how others were treated inhumanely. The discovery is unsettling, but it could explain the real modus operandi of the BWC and its cohorts. It also explains some very strange moves in health care and in ancillary companies. Certainly, it is clear that the BWC and the health care industry do not want this information to get out.

In Dr. Nichols' research and investigation into the BWC and the MCOs, he did not realize at the time that there were global entities at work whose scope went well beyond the BWC's or the State's grasp. As the investigation for the book widened, it became apparent that there was a definite reaction coming from sources outside of Ohio, sources that had the funding to thwart the process of harvesting information.

Speaking with Dr. Nichols by cell phone proved more than difficult. In fact, our phones were actually shut down, batteries drained each time we spoke, and the pattern grew more frequent. The same cell phone provider was involved. Soon, it happened when we spoke with injured workers about their cases or tried to glean information from other sources. Internet attacks were numerous and costly to our computers and to our time. Fortunately, the vital information we had was locked away from the criminally curious and that seemed to help, but it did not alleviate the problem entirely.

Finally, it became necessary to forestall any communication after a certain point was reached in order to preserve the information and not see it stolen.

Other issues arose making it difficult to continue with the investigation. Extraordinary measures had to be taken. Dr. Nichols soon realized that the ramifications of his protestations were noticed on a national, if not international level and it was no small wonder considering that he found himself right in the middle of something that was a heavily guarded secret.

Further, the investigation proves pertinent and critical linkage to the global game plan of the elite and perhaps that is why Dr. Nichols has been followed and harassed. There is a global connection behind the financial problems that were created for Dr. Nichols with his bank and stalled his financing until it drove him into the ground. The investigation proves that there is a connection with the BWC and where this world is headed, a destination that we are not supposed to know.

Fundamentally then, our world is well on its way to becoming a place envisioned by Huxley, Wells and the Rockefellers. We are seeing the manifestation of their work and in their philosophies coming to full fruition. Politicians and government officials have put these ideals into perverse practice for personal and financial gain. Together with their mentors they have implemented their concepts and taken them from the realm of science fiction into today's harsh reality. They would take our tomorrow into the surreal dimension of Big Brother on steroids, if we allow it. These people have taken the lives of countless people and are targeting millions more. Are we in danger of being targeted?

CHAPTER TEN
WORTH MORE DEAD

A disconcerting trend started to develop during this investigation that pointed to something more profound than the BWC's and MCOs' mistreatment of injured workers and while that abuse was staggering by itself, there had to be more to the problem than was visible on the surface.

Some injured workers seemed to get the treatment they needed, but there were many others with the exact same injuries that did not. In peeling back the bureau's onion skin, many other problems arose indicating that a troubling undertone was pulsing through the system and sweeping critical factors from public view.

In trying to find the one cohesive element that would expose the true infrastructure, it became clear that the labyrinth was entangled with all sorts of improprieties on dozens of levels. Discovering the connection became difficult.

Was it possible that a quota system was in place where a certain number of injured workers would receive treatment for their injuries? Perhaps when the cutoff number was met then the door closed to injured workers with the exact same injuries. It could be quite probable, but after further investigation, it appeared that concept, while it might be in operation today, seemed random. Workers that got injured at the same time with the same injuries had different outcomes within the bureau's system. Therefore, something in addition to a quota system had to be in play that was not apparent, something perhaps only discussed on the secret file levels within the bureau.

It is unlikely that the connection would be noticeable to those outside of the bureau and it would be possible to obscure the differentiation of treatment from any investigative agency, at least for a time. In the past, the chances of a group of injured workers being interviewed by independent outside sources in an attempt to glean as much information possible seemed remote. Therefore, the bureau enjoyed a level of comfort knowing that the danger of someone discovering the suspected hidden agendas that fuel the BWC would be slight. Some of that changed when Dr. Nichols decided to tackle the problems between the bureau and the injured workers causing the BWC to get more than a little paranoid.

Employees of the BWC quickly closed ranks when Dr. Nichols started filing criminal complaints against specific employees that were abusing the system and ignoring the Ohio Revised Code. He did not stop in his efforts to obtain justice for injured workers, and the bureau did not stop in throwing obstacles in his path, sometimes insurmountable ones.

Dr. Nichols felt sure that the bureau was misrepresenting their efforts to debride the festering wounds at the BWC and he was correct. There have been no sanctions or disciplinary actions that have taken place in spite of countless criminal complaints that have been filed detailing the extent of the malfeasance. Still, he knew there was a great deal more than negligence going on within the bureau. He was correct.

By interviewing several of Dr. Nichols' patients, it became apparent in the course of the investigation that the wheat and the chaff policy of the bureau was palpable, but it also revealed some other alarming dark alleys that led to a much larger and more organized network.

There are integral players like Customer Service Specialists that can game the system swinging the pendulum well into the BWC's sphere and away from the injured worker. That means that the CSS has the ability to pick and choose the information that is given to IME doctors who will determine injury, treatment and disability. Is there set criteria in the handling of individual cases?

From the disparity that is prevalent between injured workers, some criteria or parameters must be set either by the BWC or by department heads because the problem is so pervasive. The problem is too widespread to blame a few CSS personnel in swaying an examiner's opinion regarding certain injured workers or instances of specialists being too lazy to pull the entire file. Clearly, the CSS has a ridiculous amount of power when it comes to what that specialist would deem appropriate to send in a file to a review doctor or to a hearing officer. It appears likely that some files that are chosen for reviews are intact, while others have been picked through or are outright expunged and stacked against the injured worker guaranteeing a denial for treatment by the IME doctor.

Quota systems could result in more income for the BWC, and information obtained from injured workers indicates that perhaps the BWC really does have a high degree of discrimination in their care of injured workers. Is there a prejudice against former military personnel who become injured on the job?

That is certainly one possibility. Bill Durst was a veteran. In the case of Coca Cola, John Doe is a veteran and so is another injured Coca Cola worker who is being denied treatment. Other company workers seem to get better results from Coca Cola regarding work injuries. Mr. Doe's attorney, Jonathan Goodman, seems to think there might be a connection. Lewis "Rex" Whan is also a veteran, as are many of Dr. Nichols' patients who are mistreated.

Ricky Watson found out firsthand what it was like to be discriminated against because he was a veteran. At the time, he worked for River Valley Paper Company in Akron, Ohio as a truck driver and dispatcher. On a December day in 2007, Mr. Watson, 47, had to check his trailer for holes and when he tried to step down from the trailer, his foot slipped and he landed on his back. Since the trailer was parked by railroad tracks, there were large rocks in the area and unfortunately, he landed on one. The ground was cold and he laid there for a few minutes thinking he had the wind knocked out of him. He got up and walked to the office. Mr. Watson started feeling sweaty and faint, but he made it to the office.

His coworkers asked how he was doing because they had seen him fall. They were worried because Mr. Watson had grown extremely pale. He told his boss he was going to the VA hospital since he did not feel right. His wife spoke with him on the way to the VA and told him to go to a regular hospital since the accident happened at work. So he went to St. Thomas Hospital in the corporate care area.

He had to wait for two hours and while he waited he walked around the hospital corridors. Finally, he saw a doctor and an X-ray was ordered. Mr. Watson walked to the X-ray department and waited for another prolonged period before the X-ray was taken. When the doctor saw the X-ray, he told Mr. Watson he had broken his back and sent him to the emergency room where he was given a brace and some pain medication.

His manager, Jeff Robinson, allegedly did not believe Mr. Watson and told him that the company was not responsible for something that occurred during his military service. Mr. Watson was dumbfounded. Having served in the US Navy for twenty years, he had been honorably discharged ten years before the accident happened. The only trouble Mr. Watson had with his back was lumbar arthritis he acquired while working on F-14 aircraft aboard the USS Kitty Hawk and other aircraft carriers. Although he had broken an ankle and hand during his career, he never had any serious injuries to his back. Yet, Robinson felt the broken back was something that happened ten years prior and that Mr. Watson was not telling the truth.

Until the accident, Mr. Watson had never been unemployed and was always a hard-working employee. He even received favorable evaluations at the River Valley Paper Company, something that worked in his favor during the countless hearings he had to go through with the BWC. Robinson tried to claim that he was a lousy employee, but Mr. Watson had written proof he was not.

He did return to work in February and did a lot of his work at his desk. There were days when Robinson would come into his office and start screaming at Mr. Watson for no apparent reason about anything and everything trying to intimidate him to quit. One of Mr. Watson's coworkers asked why he took so much of Robinson's attitude and he said that he had been dressed down by admirals and Robinson did not scare him.

His travails with the BWC continue two years after his accident and he is fighting for all the help he can get. Like countless others, he was put into pain management and has been diagnosed as major depressive. Mr. Watson's days are filled with pain and he has struggled to get through them. He would like nothing better than to return to work. His family's finances are in chaos. It really is no coincidence that Mr. Watson is not only a veteran, but he is also an organ donor.

Perhaps the bureau labels former military personnel a bad risk in general due to recent evidence particularly among Gulf War veterans, of debilitating conditions acquired from the array of immunizations they were given or because of pre-existing conditions that were present before their discharge.

Yet, there seems to be a more definite link, which could transcend the discrimination against veterans. In doing interviews for the book, an almost macabre similarity emerged with the majority of the injured workers, especially those that were treated badly by the BWC and the MCOs. The common denominator that the majority shared was the fact that they were organ donors.

How could the BWC determine that a particular injured worker was an organ donor? After 2001, the Department of Motor Vehicles database was made available to several Ohio government agencies, and the bureau was one of them. Drivers' license information lists whether a person is an organ donor or not. It would be easy to determine in a database search that cross-referenced driver's license information and injured workers within the BWC system.

A master list could be developed and individual records could be kept on a non-public file level such as the secret file level found at the bureau. If a particular injured worker was an organ donor, their file could be flagged giving the CSS and all those with access to the data a heads up. That flag would make it easy for the CSS to make detrimental decisions to the injured worker's health and to slow the process down.

Other agencies share data, therefore, it is conceivable that they could acquire BWC information as well and that gives rise to issues involving federal privacy laws. There have been precedents where data has been sold to entities outside the government raising even more legal questions and the rights of individual citizens.

A precedent has already been established that a BWC worker accessed driver's license information for personal reasons.

An investigation conducted by the Inspector General, Thomas P. Charles and his unit conducted an investigation that revealed that Tonya

Claborn had misused state equipment and had made false statements while working as a fraud investigator at the BWC. According to the Inspector General's report, the Deputy Inspector General of the BWC and the Industrial Commission was informed of wrongdoing by Claborn, a Fraud Investigator.

Apparently, Claborn was involved in an automobile accident that happened on personal time. She had slowed to avoid a vehicle in front of her that had made a sudden stop when she was rear-ended. Information was exchanged at the scene and the driver who hit her left abruptly after giving her what turned out to be false information about his identity. When he drove off, she made note of his license plate number and later used the information and accessed the DMV records through her BWC computer to find the man's real identity. The investigative report stated, "By accessing these systems, Claborn obtained the name, vehicle identification number, driver's license number, and Social Security number of one of the drivers purportedly involved in the collision. She also conducted further research in the information systems using these data elements."[77]

This was not Claborn's first offense at the bureau. The investigation revealed that she had used bureau computers to look up credit reports on her family in 2004 and had received a written warning. Her case has been sent to the prosecutor's office. While it is important that Claborn's wrongdoing was inevitably discovered, the fact is that she was left in a position to continue her misdeeds and had access to information with which she could not be trusted.

An employee in the technology department at the BWC said that there is not enough manpower to adequately track internet usage of its employees. Point in case involved Jeff Adkins who had been viewing and accumulating pornographic material for years using his BWC computer.[78] Adkins even asked for a private cubicle, which he received, and allowed him to continue his uninterrupted viewing for a very long time. The bureau did not catch Adkins' activities for years even though he was one of the highest users of the internet. This is because inadequate tracking software was in place to detect improper surfing. One supervisor that found the sites Adkins was viewing were very disturbing and he regretted not asking about the content before viewing the site.

The Watchdog report listed some of Adkins' activities:

"Visited non-work related Web sites, including several that were sexually graphic, for hours at a time. He visited at least one adult site 67 of the 106 days he reported for work between May 5 and Oct. 15.

---

[77] State of Ohio Office of Inspector General's June 26, 2009 investigation report.
[78] CantonRep.com January 26, 2009 Report: Ohio Worker's porn surfing goes undetected by Andrew Welsh-Huggins

"Opened and stored at least 318 sexually oriented movies, 11 adult audio files and more than 1,200 adult photos. Sent and received dozens of e-mails connected to his volunteer job as technology director for his church.

"Used his work computer to visit Web sites for aspiring writers and spent "excessive amounts of time" sending instant messages, blogging and other writing related to making films, writing church plays and sexually oriented fiction stories."[79]

In spite of some remedies that were put in place ex post facto, it is difficult to police employees' internet usage, especially if they use co-workers computers.

In another incident, a class action lawsuit was filed that alleges that two employees of the Ohio Department of Public Safety and Bureau of Motor Vehicles broke the law when they allowed the sale of drivers' information on state databases. Court documents filed in US District Court in Ohio stated that names, addresses, and drivers' license numbers were sold to PublicData. It is not known if organ donor information was sold with the rest of the information, but the opportunity was there. Apparently, hundreds of thousands of names and corresponding information were sold to PublicData, which in turn resold the information to Shadowsoft.

Charles Lester, an attorney associated with Eric Deters' law firm, is handling the case for the plaintiffs. He stated, "Anyone can go get that information, all you have to do is pay a fee – there is no vetting process that stops you. If you wanted to go get information about the judge in the case I could go online and get it!"[80]

The class action suit seeks to prevent the State of Ohio from selling information and for the State to retrieve information that is already out in cyberspace, if that is possible. Yet, the damage is done and proves that information can be a powerful and profitable tool. These incidents prove that it is possible to use government data and to harvest considerable amounts of information on individual citizens whether done individually or done as an agency protocol.

There has been data selling originating from within the BWC as well. In 2008, a BWC employee allegedly sold names, social security numbers and private information of injured workers to a private investigator. Supposedly, identity theft was not the reason for the sale. The private investigator bought the information on 49 injured workers, but his reasons for obtaining the information were not made clear. The case went to the Cuyahoga County Prosecutor's Office.[81]

---

[79] http://watchdog.ohio.gov/investigations/2008298.pdf
[80] Lawyers and Settlements.com : Ohio Drivers Miffed by Sale of Private Info, July 11, 2009 by Brenda Craig
[81] PI Buzz, January 5, 2008: Ohio BWC Worker Allegedly Admits to Selling Data to Private Investigator, by Jimmie Mesis

This case proves that BWC workers do have access to pertinent information and can use it in a covert manner without much oversight on the bureau's part, but it is just as likely that the information is viewed and used by countless BWC workers through the course of the day. Access to the DMV records makes it much easier for the bureau and its employees to know which injured workers are organ donors and could easily adjust their treatment strategies accordingly.

In forming this theory, it is essential to look at the rising number of deaths of injured workers during the time they are involved in the Workers' Compensation process. Non-injury deaths in 2002 were approximately 2100 as opposed to 8,108 in 2006. That is a significant rise, a rise for which the BWC has chosen not to give an explanation. Since DMV records became available to the bureau after 2001, perhaps it is possible to see why the numbers jumped four times what they were in 2002.

The BWC joined in a curious partnership with SXC that started in November 1, 2009. Although SXC manages pharmaceutical information and various aspects of drug treatment, it also is involved in transplants. Ohio, like other states, has a long list of people waiting for transplants because there are not enough organ donors to meet the demand.

If we look at the BWC data concerning Dr. Nichols' patients, we can see a penchant for dragging out the claim, particularly on injured workers who are organ donors. It has been common for these claims to extend four years and beyond. That situation alone normally can push the injured worker into the pain management scenario and as the last chapter proved, that course of action carries with it a high mortality rate.

Pain management has grown more popular in recent years with the bureau and that could explain the high numbers of non-injury deaths that have occurred since 2002, but it also shows that the bulk of those injured workers were most likely victims of delayed treatment and quite possibly they were organ donors. If we use Dr. Nichols' patients as a control group that seems quite likely.

Government agencies are getting into the business of organ harvesting and are funding groups that actively seek donors and often times rush to harvest organs even while the donor is still alive. The House of Representatives drew up an act called the 2004 Organ Donation and Recovery Improvement Act, which provides grants to hospitals and groups that work at procuring organs. The act addressed the Uncontrolled Donors after Cardiac Death. There is a new trend now that presumes consent. According to the Uniform Anatomical Gift Act, it states that any lack of refusal or specific consent does not preclude donation. The burden supposedly falls on the next of kin, but since time is of the essence in organ harvesting, there is room for concern.

The US law is clear that any organ donation must come from expressed consent, and presumed consent is supposed to be illegal. However, that is not the case in countries like Spain where presumed consent is the norm. That movement is gaining popularity in Europe and several countries are now considering changing their organ donation laws. Some US legislators are working to drastic changes in our organ donor laws.

For instance, in the UK, Gordon Brown seriously considered revamping organ donor laws to mark everyone as a potential donor. Experts worry that would make people resistant to medical care in general for fear that their organs might be targeted. Perry and Gloria Marteney felt very strongly that would be the case here in the US and neither one is an organ donor, two of a small number of Dr. Nichols' patients who are not. Yet, there are experts that insist that countless lives could be saved by instituting presumed consent citing that very few people actually donate their organs, while the list grows for those in need of transplants. There are movements here in the US trying to change the law to presumed consent as well.

Steve Forbes mentioned in his August 24, 2009 column that something should be done such as monetary incentives for organ donors such as having funeral costs paid for or insurance benefits for those who agree to become donors. Forbes suggested a cheaper approach would be to waive driver's license fees for anyone agreeing to become a donor.[82] That might help the situation, but not immediately. Until then, the black market and illegal organ harvesting could thrive giving those involved great remuneration.

With non-work related deaths rising yearly at the BWC, the potential for remuneration is significant, if the harvester can see $100,000 per corpse, and with demand quite high, and too few donors, it is a seller's market. Over 1 million tissue transplants are done every year, and although one corpse can yield enough material for several transplants, the demand is enormous and the quantity of donors always falls short. Organ harvesters are always looking for a new supply chain and are hoping to find amenable helpers in acquiring new donors.

Within the BWC, there is a group of people that are in a pivotal position to broach the subject of organ donation to injured workers who suffer catastrophic accidents. A Catastrophic Nurse Advocate helps severely injured workers through rehabilitation and presumably acts as an activist for the worker to make sure that the best possible treatment is given. The CNA works as an intercessor with the BWC and the MCOs and tries to keep the communication channels open. CNA's make hospital and home visits to injured workers and are in a unique position to get to know the worker on a much more personal basis and to understand their needs, which develops a different dynamic to their relationship. Communication about organ donation could be mentioned or fostered. Due to severe injuries, some injured workers are in need of organ transplants and the advocate helps with the care and monitoring of the injured

---

[82] Why Should They Die? Steve Forbes, August 24, 2009 Forbes.com

worker. In their distinctive position, they can clearly understand the need for donors and the family has an even greater understanding. In trying to interview Catastrophic Nurse Advocates about the organ donor realities, the bureau said there was no way to contact them.

It has been a topic of great debate worldwide that is predominantly confined to medical circles, which concerns the use of less than perfect organs. With the demands for transplants so high, quality organs are sometimes hard to find and so transplant surgeons go with the organs they can acquire. Often that presents problems as it did for Corporal Matthew Millington of the United Kingdom.

Due to a lung disease, Corporal Millington was in desperate need of a double lung transplant, which he received. However, at the time of the transplant he was unaware that the donor was a heavy smoker, one that smoked from 30 to 50 cigarettes per day. Although the transplant was successful, within the year a cancerous growth was spotted on a lung and he subsequently died from lung cancer. His family was completely devastated and had no idea that inferior organs would be used.

Doctors defend the use of less desirable organs because it does give the patients more time, and they say that organs were working normally in the donor. Therefore it is worth the risk. Even injured worker organs would be highly marketable since there is no real way to meet the need of one million people waiting for organs throughout the world.

Demand is so high for donors that sometimes tissue banks desperately seek donors who have just died. A monumental case in New Jersey and New York disclosed the desperation within the transplant industry to acquire as many post mortem donors as possible.

The case received international attention because the body of the well-known author, commentator and host of Masterpiece Theater, Alistair Cooke, was among those bodies hijacked so that bones and tissues could be harvested.

His daughter had no idea when she phoned a New York mortuary to pick up her father's body that her father's remains, riddled with cancer, would in effect be stolen. She assumed the body was cremated and never thought anything else. Apparently, Cooke's body was among countless bodies that were used to help supply tissue, organs and bones to Regeneration Technologies, which operates in Florida

In Cooke's case, RTI was looking for long bones and under the direction of Michael Mastromarino, a former maxillofacial surgeon turned harvester, Cooke's legs were sawed off and sold to RTI. Mastromarino operated in a New York funeral home, with the approval of the FDA and using a license provided by the New York State Department of Health.

Offering morticians $1000 per corpse, Mastromarino found willing funeral director steady supply of involuntary donors. He paid a nurse to harvest tissues, organs and bones for approximately $200-$300 per corpse in addition to a regular salary. Business boomed and the work was steady.

Several problems arose at the outset that Mastromarino took care of immediately. Many of the corpses of course never gave their consent for their organs or tissues to be harvested and neither did their next of kin. As in the case of Alistair Cooke, the deceased's family did not know anything about it. To satisfy the law, donation documents were forged using fictitious names of "family members." Not all states require that kind of documentation. In Ohio, all that is needed is for the donor's drivers' license to show that they had opted to become organ donors. Once the donation form is signed when getting an Ohio license, the license is labeled and that is all that is required unless the driver is under 18 years old. Therefore, it would be even easier in Ohio to carry out this kind of operation.

Eventually, the funeral home was sold and the new owners were shocked at the harvesting operation that was taking place in a secret room of the mortuary. They called the police. As the investigation progressed, it became clear that many of the bodies that were used in the harvest were diseased and that the chance of infecting the recipients of tissues and bones was quite high. A recall of tissues that had already gone out took place and alarms sounded in attorneys' offices throughout the country as recipients and members of the involuntary donors' families filed suit.

RTI claimed that the risk of infection was slight because of their extraordinary process of cleaning the tissues and bones. Nevertheless, panic hit.

The black market continues to flourish and the harvesting has been so intense that some hospitals are not waiting for patients to die before the harvest begins. As people live longer and body parts wear out, the need is even greater and some harvesters are very quick to supply the necessary parts.

In 2003, a report appeared in The Courier Mail that detailed the organ harvesting of kidneys from homeless people. Russian surgeons taking part in the harvest were paid $40,000 per kidney. Having total disregard for the involuntary donor, one anonymous surgeon showed his contempt by saying the people, "are done for anyway, maybe they could live another three or four days."[83]

Some doctors, like Dr. John Shea have stated that "the less dead a person is the better," when it comes to donating organs.[84] Shea, the Medical Advisor to Campaign Life Coalition, says the ethics and the nature of organ harvesting are not just inherent to Russia, but are a worldwide concern.

---

[83] LifeSiteNews.com—September 9, 2003, Russian Surgeons Removing Organs Saying Patients Almost Dead Anyways
[84] ibid

A Colorado coroner claimed that a hospital had removed organs from a patient who was not yet dead. Mark Young, the coroner for Montrose County, Colorado, ruled the death a homicide and held Montrose Memorial and St Mary's hospitals responsible in the death of William Rardin, who was a registered organ donor. He shot himself and was declared brain dead. Young said the hospitals did not use "acceptable medical standards" to determine if Rardin was actually dead.

According to Young, Rardin's liver, kidneys, and pancreas were removed while he was still alive. Standards for determining death can vary from hospital to hospital. For this problem to be resolved, a mandated set of standards should be implemented.

Most people would be appalled to know that according to one Australian doctor most organ donations are carried out on the living. Dr. James Tibballs has strong concerns about organ donations carried out before the donors are dead. He cites the differences of standards regarding the actuality of brain death and cardiac death. In brain death, blood flow to the brain must have ceased completely, but there have been many cases where donors awake on the operating table just after incisions are made. This is due to the fact that blood pressure rises and can be instrumental in resuscitating a person who has purportedly died. Citing the rush to harvest organs before they deteriorate, doctors might push the envelope.

There are some controversial arguments surfacing about the legitimacy of brain death. Dr. Paul Byrne, a neonatologist said, "Brain death was concocted, it was made up in order to get organs.[85] It was never based on science." He does seem to have a point. Still, cardiac deaths have also had their miraculous cases as well. In France, one man who had suffered cardiac arrest for approximately ninety minutes and was on the operating table when he suddenly started breathing and his pupils dilated after the incision was made. Today, the man is alive and well.

While it is felt that brain dead donors have no sense of pain, the practice in harvesting now is to use anesthesia because it prohibits movement in the donor and according to one source, makes it less difficult for the doctors and nurses involved in the harvesting. It also ensures that any recovery on the part of the donor is obliterated.

As the need for organs continues in our society, there will always be a chance for an abuse of the system. There is no better example than the news from China about the torture and incarceration of Falun Gong practitioners whose organs have been harvested by the thousands. Falun Gong is considered to be a religious movement that started in China around 1992 and has grown to 70 million followers in China and approximately 100 million worldwide. The

---

[85] October 21, 2008 LifeSiteNews.com: Melbourne Doctor: Most Donors Still Alive when Organs are Removed by Kathleen Gilbert

Chinese government started rounding up Falun Gong followers and now has them imprisoned in 36 concentration camps throughout China. Those death camps are used for organ harvesting. The prisoners are examined and the healthy ones are executed so their organs can be harvested.

Records indicate that somewhere between 7,000 and 8,000 kidney transplants are done each year in China with 99 percent of the kidneys coming from executed prisoners. The death camps are a veritable super market for organs. The authorities take blood samples so that they can get perfect matches for the organs that they sell. The Chinese government, in one of their finest demonstrations of capitalism, sells the organs around the world to the highest bidder.

This is not something novel in China, but something that was implemented in the days of Mao Tse Tung after the CIA helped put him into power following World War II. Initially, the changes Mao instituted were part of the great "Chinese experiment" promoted by the Rockefeller Foundation, the CIA and other US government agencies. The goal was a massive culling of the population starting with citizens who were considered less desirable. The Falun Gong practitioners are modern day evidence to this protracted culling. When you consider the tens of millions of people killed in China since Mao took the country by the throat and the legacy he left, David Rockefeller's statements about the situation are at best frightening.

He said, "Whatever the price of the Chinese Revolution it is obviously succeeded, not only in producing more efficient and dedicated administration but also in fostering high morale and community of purpose. The social experiment in China under Chairman Mao's leadership is one of the most important and successful in history."[86]

Supposedly, the Chinese experiment is to be used as a blueprint for population containment and global health care. We are already seeing the effects.

In New York for example, the wait for a kidney is eight to ten years, and in New Jersey, the wait is four to five years, but for kidneys coming from China, the wait is approximately only one week. Many people travel to China from all over the world to get kidneys and other organs because it is much quicker and in many cases cheaper. Some recipients are unaware that the organs are coming from donors executed to fill their need. According to the Canadian government, which has actively investigated the situation, executed prisoners cannot account for the entire rise in organ transplants. During the six year period from 2000 to 2005, there have been 41,500 transplants that cannot be explained.

---

[86] New York Times, David Rockefeller's Opinion Piece, August 10, 1973,

Chinese Hospitals freely advertise their transplant capabilities and fees, but offer no real explanation as to the origination of the organs used in transplants.

An alleged organ trafficking ring in New York was also discovered, which was purportedly run by a rabbi who charged as much as $160,000 per kidney. The rabbi had contacts in Israel who helped him acquire kidneys for people in the US. The group allegedly placed ads in Israeli papers asking people to sell their kidneys. When responses did not match demand, Russian immigrants were supposedly coerced into giving up their kidneys by the Israelis involved in the ring. Mount Sinai Hospital in New York allegedly handled at least one transplant. The donor was flown from Israel, paid for his services and met the recipient of the kidney at Mount Sinai claiming to be his cousin. Although the hospital stated that it did get some background information, they were not detectives and it as not its obligation to challenge the veracity of the donor. The surgeries took place and the trafficking ring had a handsome payday. According to the man who sold his kidney through the rabbi's network, the hospital must have known the situation, but did not challenge him.

There are other reports throughout the country of these kinds of transactions, and we are experiencing a pattern of sorts that warns us of a very dangerous future. We are already seeing that medicine has changed its views in the past forty years, from psychiatry to general practice, there is a growing delineation between the salvageable patient and the dispensable one. The medical and insurance industries have a new battle cry in this troubling shift in patient care. The "Greater Good" is the term used most often to further a particular agenda, one that has ominous consequences.

Organ donation in its purest sense is almost perfect charity, one person's gift of life to another, but while that might be true on the part of conscious donors who make the brave decision to donate their organs upon death, it is not true of many of the organizations in operation today.

The wheat and the chaff philosophy of the BWC is not original to the bureau, but was developed by groups of powerful people like the Rockefellers, who funded the very first studies in organ transplants in the early 1900's.

One of the Rockefellers' scientists, Alexis Carrel, was a French surgeon who worked for their foundation from 1906 until he retired in 1939. Carrel did extensive research in suturing techniques on blood vessels and organ transplants, and won the Nobel Prize for Medicine in 1912.

The route medicine has taken was mapped out decades ago and we are seeing those plans reach their maturation in ominous ways. The world has rushed towards the disposability of some human beings, either the sick, the poor or those that are a burden on society who do not have a vital role, the useless eaters as the elite would call them, have made a hit list.

With some doctors, that list started years ago. A specific case stands out regarding a woman in Portland, Oregon, a mother and grandmother who was hospitalized with an exacerbation of Multiple Sclerosis. MS is a waxing and waning illness that attacks the myelin sheath around the nerves in the brain. Often MS patients can have quite normal stretches, but there are times that the disease can become more pronounced. This woman was in the hospital during one of the more difficult periods of MS and one day she could not swallow.

Apparently the doctor notified the woman's family and informed them of the situation. Her family arrived with the woman's young grandson. They came to visit her and to say goodbye. The boy was no more than eight or nine. He held her hand and spoke to her and she was glad he was there. The doctor came in and looked at her chart, then gave the woman a cursory exam. A patient in the next bed along with her family were appalled at what happened next. The doctor said that because the woman could no longer swallow that it was time for her to be relieved of her suffering. Of course the boy starting to cry as did the woman in the other bed, who at 102 years old worried she might be next. Due to the fact that MS does wax and wane, it was quite possible for the woman to recover in the next few days or even hours with treatment, but she was not given that option nor consulted.

The doctor injected the woman and the boy watched as his grandmother's body twitched. The doctor turned to him and stated that it was just muscle spasms and she was feeling no pain. In a few moments she was gone, much to the amazement and to the horror of the witnesses. The doctor managed to free up a bed, but left a nightmare not only for the family but also for the others in the room.

Euthanasia laws have gained ground as have assisted suicides, but in the end, each one of us loses because we have lost the moral compass we acquired at birth. The prospect of health care worldwide has turned ghoulish and its foundation was conceived in the late 1800's and early 1900's. Promulgated and funded by the elite, today's health care is their vision, but need not be ours. However, as economics play an even greater role in the decision making process in Washington, the average person, like the people who built this country from the ground up, will be considered expendable, disposable and a burden on the rest of society. The new health care in this country is the direct result of a few deciding the fate for the masses.

Dr. Nichols' fight with the BWC and the fight of a few others cannot result in a victory for the injured workers abused by the bureau unless enough people join them to raise voices loud enough and bring enough attention to the corruption that is present there today. When enough people join the fight that cannot be squelched, cannot be driven into the ground financially and cannot be intimidated by the organized criminals within the bureau, then there will be true justice and swift and appropriate treatment for the injured workers.

Yet, the fight is beyond the BWC and Ohio. It is quickly becoming a global issue that has been carefully concealed. Under our very noses, people are being victimized. Their medical treatment is geared not towards healing, but rather towards feeding a self-perpetuating system. It is quickly becoming a world where the best medical care is only given to a select few and the rest of us are expendable. Our value lies in the market rate for organs and beyond that we are useless.

The atrocities that are happening within health care around the world are no different than what we see happening in the third world where countless souls are lost to famine, to poverty and to revolts and civil unrest. In a sense, health care has created a paradoxical third world within itself, where the haves get treatment and the have not's get substandard care. Like what is happening in Rwanda, we are seeing the culling of people where guns are not used but rather prescriptions and scalpels to achieve a goal.

What Henry Kissinger said in 1974 could easily apply to the health care system designed by him and his cohorts. He said, "Depopulation should be the highest priority of foreign policy towards the third world." Social Darwinism has been applied by the Rockefellers, the Council on Foreign Relations, the Trilateral Commission and the Bilderbergs on the masses.

In effect, those caught up in the BWC can expect to be divided much like those people in the death camps of World War II. The people that are reasonably healthy and can be an asset to society line up on the right for treatment and those that do not meet an established criteria line up on the left, which becomes the end of the line.

The same is true for people that have private insurance. These conglomerates operate in the same way. They pay a great deal for positive publicity, advertise about their tremendous benefits, but when it comes time to take care of the sick or injured, excuses, delays and abuse are piled on to the insured at a time when that person is down.

The game and how it is played is the same. The people that run these organizations are well-chosen and have the very best connections to a network of greed, murder and corruption. The very nature of health care is aberrant today and without our banding together, we can be assured of more victims so numerous it would be difficult to count.

CHAPTER ELEVEN
VICTORY IN DEFEAT

Dr. Nichols has been involved in countless cases where the abuse of the injured worker seemed unfathomable. From the atrocities that have happened to patients like Bill Durst and Perry Marteney and a myriad of others, to the ridiculous nature of some IME examinations, Dr. Nichols has seen it all, but he is still astonished at the degree of the corruption and duplicity. Recently, he attended an IME exam with Ricky Watson to see how it was performed and to serve as a witness. When the doctor examined Mr. Watson's reflexes, he used a stethoscope, not a mallet. The exam was so brief and unprofessional that it left both Nichols and Watson wondering about the competence of the doctor.

Without advocates like Dr. Nichols, it is hard for injured workers to get an unbiased examination and all too often well renowned hospitals are part of the problem. There seems to be a condescending approach to the treatment of injured workers and perhaps one of the main reasons is that the average education of the Ohio worker is a sixth grade education. In the eyes of the BWC, MCOs, doctors and hospitals, injured workers can be viewed as substandard, and not intelligent enough to realize they are being hoodwinked. With that arrogance there is a mindset of Them versus Us that brings with it a despicable prejudice and a predictable negative outcome.

The people engaged in the Workers' Compensation arena have an unfair advantage over injured workers. Trying to recover from devastating work related injuries, the financial fallout and psychological problems that can ensue preoccupy the injured worker and often weaken their resolve and their ability to fight back. It is not an unfair observation to suggest that the BWC relies on that. Discounting the injured worker's worth is a major problem within the system and all too often bruised and battered workers give up the fight dying either literally or figuratively.

There are cases that bring hope and serve as examples that injured workers could be victorious in their battles to overcome the bureaucratic byproducts of the BWC. One remarkable case is that of Sarah Shick.

Ms. Shick was working at her third job, which was at a bar in the Cleveland area. She was decorating the bar for the 4th of July. Beautiful and bright, Ms. Shick, 26, had a positive future. She was a college student with a cumulative grade point average of 3.91 and well on her way to making a good life. She had a loving boyfriend, supportive family and life was good until something went horribly wrong at work.

Behind the bar was a trap door, which led to where the beer and other bar materials were kept. When the door was open, the bar owner's policy was to have employees holler, "Door's open." There were never any barricades around the trap door and according to Ms. Shick, there were no reprimands given to employees that failed to alert the other staff about the door. While she worked, no one yelled that the door was open and therefore she had no way of knowing she was headed for disaster. Ms. Shick had just finished putting decorations around the television when she fell backwards into the trap door. She fell so hard that she bounced up and then landed several feet below, hitting her head and landing on her back. Ms. Shick was the sixth person within three years to fall through the trapdoor in the bar's tainted and OSHA challenged history.

Stunned, she lay on the concrete floor and was having trouble breathing, apparently she had the wind knocked out of her. Her injuries were a concussion, neck sprain, and a right shoulder sprain, a fracture of the T-12 vertebra, right SI joint injury, and thoracic and lumbar sprains. Her liver was damaged and she had to take medication to regulate its proper function.

Ms. Shick's problems had only begun. She went through Workers' Compensation for her claim and she tried to work with her employer, who had a history of ducking his responsibilities. In other injuries that happened at the bar, he lied to those workers who were injured claiming he did not have Workers' Compensation insurance and the employees did not realize that the insurance was mandatory for all employers in Ohio.

Once Ms. Shick got her claim started, she decided to move against the owner legally. The bar owner had been to law school and knew what was bearing down on him. He bolted and skipped town. He tried to sell the bar on the sly, but Ms. Shick and her lawyer found out from the bar's manager and they were successful in barring the sale. Following the sale of the bar equipment and miscellaneous supplies, eventually she got a small settlement from the owner, and from Workers' Compensation because the bar owner did not follow any OSHA safety guidelines.

Throughout her therapy, Ms. Shick was part of the MCO process with Sheakley. She had a fairly good case manager by the name of Betsy H. who walked her through the process and seemed truly interested in helping her. Betsy worked on her claim for about thirty-six months. Betsy tried to help Ms. Shick through the pain management process even suggesting acupuncture, which surprised Ms. Shick and her doctors as well, especially since Betsy, an MCO case manager, suggested it. It was not long after that that Betsy disappeared and Ms. Shick had no idea what happened to her. She called Sheakley and asked about her and was referred to another case manager who informed her that Betsy took a job closer to home. Ms. Shick thought it was very odd because Betsy always called to inform her of any changes with Sheakley and the BWC claims process.

Having trouble with muscle spasms and pain in her lower back, Ms. Shick was told to consider having radio frequency obliteration[87] done to kill the nerve causing the problem. She did her research about the procedure and went to the celebrated Cleveland Clinic to have it done. Trying to keep up with her studies, Ms. Shick wanted to do her part in her recovery because she felt it was her job, since she could not work.

Following the radio frequency obliteration, she returned home. She began having severe muscle spasms in her hip, which was pulled down and forward at the same time. The spasms were so terrible and painful that her body was contorting with them. Ms. Shick called the Cleveland Clinic and was told that the nerve was dying and that it would be a few days for it to resolve itself. However, the pain got worse as did the spasms, so Ms. Shick contacted the clinic again and they agreed to see her.

After being examined, she was told that she now had severe bursitis in the hip and it was suggested that she have steroid injections. Apparently, bursitis was a possible side effect from the radio frequency obliteration.

The Memorial Day weekend approached and she made an appointment to go in for the injections on the following Tuesday. She had just finished a term paper, turned it in and expected to take a two week break before starting summer classes. Ms. Shick did not anticipate any problems with the injections, and hoped that it would eliminate the spasms and pain she was having so she could focus on her studies.

When she arrived for her appointment, she told the doctor that she needed something for the spasms before having the injections done. The nurse looked at her chart and agreed along with other staff members, but her doctor, Dr. Cheng did not agree and proceeded without medicating her.

She received six injections of steroids and lidocaine. The injections were horrifically painful, so much so that an Operation Room technician came over to her and held her hand and encouraged her throughout the process. When the doctor completed the injections, she got up to go home, but her legs and

---

[87] Radio Frequency Obliteration uses heat to destroy or diminish the nerve's capacity to emit pain signals to the brain.

back felt tingly and numb. Told she could drive herself home after the procedure, she reevaluated that and had someone come and get her. When she got home, she went to bed and fell asleep for approximately four hours.

When she woke up, she tried to get up to go to the bathroom and discovered she had difficulty walking. Two more hours elapsed and she could not walk at all. Her boyfriend had to carry her to the bathroom. Understandably upset, he called the Cleveland Clinic and asked what they had done to Ms. Shick. By this time, she was in severe pain, but the clinic advised her to double up on her pain medication and muscle relaxers. Concerned the extra medication would kill her; she took another pain pill, but halved the muscle relaxer. Her condition did not improve and in fact deteriorated.

Her boyfriend rushed her to the clinic where she stayed for eight hours. An X-ray was ordered, but the physician who performed the steroid injections refused to come and see her. He told the Emergency Room physician to send her home. According to Ms. Shick, the ER doctor did not want to override the doctor's decision because he had performed the injections and thought it was his call.

Ms. Shick protested and said that it was not safe for her to go home because she could not walk or take care of herself. The ER doctor finally agreed and admitted her to the hospital for 24 hours. During that time her roommate died and she had an awful night.

She was seen by a pain management doctor who said she was suffering from fibromyalgia,[88] which should not impact her ability to walk. The hospital seemed to use a strong offensive with Ms. Shick and they did so with a vengeance.

Five psychologists were brought in to talk to her and she could see that there was a concerted effort going on to make her believe that her paralysis was all in her head. Yet, that would not explain why, upon physical examination, it was discovered she had drop foot, a good indication that paralysis was part of the problem. The clinic then sent in the head of the neurology department to refute that. She took Ms. Shick's foot and pushed it down and told her it moved and that she could do it. At that point, the doctor told her she was suffering from some sort of convergence disorder, which is taking psychological problems and turning them into physical maladies.

Ms. Shick has a positive personality and is well adjusted, which seemed to work against her in the hospital. When she first arrived, she was not giving the proper pain medication. Then after she was given medication, she was considered too euphoric because of pain medication. In actuality she was just being naturally positive. The nurses on her floor stood up for her and protested

---

[88] The Mayo Clinic definition of fibromyalgia is "a chronic condition characterized by widespread pain in your muscles, ligaments and tendons, as well as fatigue and multiple tender points-places on your body where slight pressure causes pain."

to the doctor saying that her entire family was positive and that Ms. Shick was trying to make the best of a nasty situation.

The doctor who had done the steroid injections was pressured by one of his colleagues to visit Ms. Shick and he finally made a brief appearance eight days into her hospitalization. He told her that he hoped she knew that her problems were not his fault. His offensive and belligerent attitude was hard for her to take.

She stayed in the hospital for two weeks, but her condition did not improve. Unable to go home, she ended up at the Menorah Park Center for Senior Living, a nursing home. At 26, she was the youngest resident. It must have been terribly frustrating for her to be in a nursing home. Her future looked bleak, but Ms. Shick never gave up. She utilized the aquatics center attached to Menorah Park and found that water exercises benefitted her greatly. Not able to return to her summer classes, Ms. Shick put all of her energies into getting better.

Her trials in getting treatments paid for were much like the other injured workers. If she had not had the settlement money, she would not have been able to stay at the nursing home and get treatment. The BWC denied her claims and the whole hearing process ensued, but she ultimately prevailed. In trying to get help through her MCO, she was at least vindicated when her case worker said when she went to the Cleveland Clinic "They did something wrong and they hurt you." For that privilege, the clinic billed her $45,000.

Able to return home, but still in need of mobility, Ms. Shick thought about a wheelchair, but did not want to go that route. She preferred something "Cool and creative rather than sad and tragic." So she chose a Segway scooter, similar to the ones used in Paul Blart Mall Cop. Using a wheelchair was very painful for Ms. Shick because her neck, shoulder and arm muscles ached to the point she could not sleep at night. With the Segway she has a greater degree of mobility and could meet people on eye level.

Reflecting on her experience with Workers' Compensation, Ms. Shick said, "If I have times I feel suicidal, I can't imagine people who don't have my education handle it. I have to fight everyday to keep my health."

She was given a chance to address the BWC and delivered an eloquent indictment of its system. Ms. Shick said, "I want to start by thanking you for honoring me with your attention. Almost three years ago exactly I was working two jobs to try return to college when I was setting up for an event at the bar I worked at. As I was putting up the final decorations I fell backwards through an open trap door, down a flight of stairs and on to a concrete floor. I sustained many injuries, several of which took time to become apparent. I was the sixth person in three years to fall through that trap door. I regularly told the owner of the risk, but despite my warnings, nothing was done to fix it.

"As I started my recovery, I was very overwhelmed and confused by the BWC process, and realized that I would need assistance in navigating the system. I made a point to connect with my case workers at BWC and my MCO, but quickly found I needed to hire a lawyer to be able to receive my full rights, such a fair financial compensation and appropriate medical care. I had gone into the system believing that it was a relatively benevolent organization with the simple goal of doing what it takes to get me healthy, functioning, and able to return to work. In return for this assistance, I approached my recovery with the mindset that it was my new job and that I must work hard and be dedicated to hold up my part of this deal.

"Despite my hard work, I learned that there was no one person who was taking a fair and complete look at my case. I had to become my own medical manager, a task that is beyond the skills and energy level of most injured workers I encounter. If I stack my files regarding my case on the ground, they are over two and a half feet tall. At nearly every step of the way I have had to fight my MCO for coverage of services that were clearly medically relevant. I have been to the industrial commission for so many hearings that the security guard and I have become friends (he always has a peppermint for me). Frequently, the denial and appeal process delayed care in ways that stalled my recovery and even resulted in physical regression.

"In trying to hold up my end of the deal in working towards recovery, I have even paid out of pocket for recommended treatments, medications and assistive devices that has added up to over $10,000.

"The denials that I faced with my vocational rehab (which was medically suspended), made me even more scared about returning to work. I was bullied by my MCO to join their Voc Rehab program and threatened with 'many denials and an uphill battle' if I went with the Voc Rehab vendor of my choice. This highly unethical conversation was recorded and turned over to the Bureau. The way vocational rehab is set up now feels like an assembly line with little individual flexibility. This **should** be a process of hope and progress that creates confident and capable workers who are not so rushed that they risk re-injury.

"One of the most detrimental denials I have faced was the denial of the emotional care I requested. I understand that there is a social stigma against mental health care, but within the BWC, I was shocked that it took me three years of requests to get the care I needed. What could have been initially treated with some counseling and short term anti-depressants has now lead to crippling depression and anxiety that has been amended on my claim. Isn't there something that can be done before a person is further disabled by what is a natural result of trauma and chronic pain?

"I have fought desperately to recover, even after losing my ability to walk after surgical complications. Yet, I am one of the lucky ones. I have friends on BWC who have lost their homes because of the financial impacts of their injuries. I have known of too many relationships destroyed by the stress of being in medical limbo without much hope (and even my own relationship has struggled to survive). I have watched a friend confide in her MCO case manager only to have that confidence manipulated in order to deny treatment. I have personally had to talk three different people out of committing suicide because they can't get the care and support they need.

"I know that you all face a daunting task in managing a system like this. I also know that there are many other states with far more successful systems. The constant denial and hearing process costs the state far more money than listening to the treating physicians and injured workers and allowing medically relevant care. The lawyers are struggling to protect their clients as they are inundated with constant denials. The greed that is present in this MCO system is not just costing money, it is costing lives.

"Through this experience I have encountered phenomenal dedication and caring people, from lawyers to caseworkers and health care providers. Their passion and skill should not be diminished by the corruption that now so pervasive in the BWC system. Please understand, we are not just injured workers, we are mothers, friends, cousins, and want to get back to being productive human beings. In your challenging task of organizing and running such a behemoth of a system, please remember that it is your obligation to protect your fellow human beings on the most basic levels."

Her speech seemed to have no impact on the bureau, which continues operating in the same way. Ms. Shick's case is nothing new to the bureau and cases like hers are replayed into hundreds of thousands every year. The bureau is not interested in checking on her status to see how she is doing and neither is her MCO. She is on her own.

Ms. Shick used her education to help fight her own battle and organized the mountain of forms and letters she received, which helped her lawyer in her case. She stayed on top of the situation in spite of her pain knowing that she had to help herself. Dr. Nichols said that injured workers are "Sucked into the abyss they can't get out." Ms. Shick was obviously one of the exceptions. Her age and her education helped her to overcome the avalanche of problems and her indomitable spirit will undoubtedly lead her to a bright future.

She has been accepted into law school and is taking classes part-time feeling that a law degree will help her to support herself and the sedentary nature of the job will be easier for her disability. Had she not won her settlements, had she not believed in herself, had she not challenged the medical and insurance professionals, the outcome would not have been as positive. Ms. Shick is an exception, blessed to have faced the enemy with her spirit intact and more importantly, came out alive.

Other injured Ohio workers have also found a victory of sorts. Dr. Nichols has a patient whose mother supposedly is in an influential position working for Rush Limbaugh. When her son injured his back, the claim went the same way as many injured worker claims until Dr. Nichols told the case manager about the Rush connection. He knew what the outcome would be and he was right. This man's treatments are not delayed and in many cases seem to be expedited. Injured workers without the ever important six degrees of separation have to fight for their victory even though they are written off.

One particular case concerns Alan Kirkman, whose case was more cut and dried and certainly lacked the ambiguity of what the BWC has attached to back injuries. Nevertheless, it was a case fraught with bureaucratic bunk.

Mr. Kirkman was working for a temporary service that had him stationed at Colfor Manufacturing. He was working on a cold forging press when the die exploded. A piece of shrapnel was shot through his left elbow and into his left side lodging just millimeters from his spine. According to Dr. Nichols, the shrapnel came close to severing the aorta.

Amazingly, Mr. Kirkman stayed on his feet. His foreman saw what happened, grabbed him and ran him to the office. Mr. Kirkman said there was so much blood it "looked like a horror movie." It was estimated that he lost about three pints of blood and he thought he would bleed to death before the ambulance arrived.

After a week, he was finally able to get out of his hospital bed. His recovery was slow and his fight with the bureau even slower. The most significant battles came with the IME doctors who supposedly examined him and their findings were some of the most outrageous that Dr. Nichols has seen.

Mr. Kirkman had an appointment with Dr. Paul T. Scheatzle of Bailey Rehabilitation for an IME examination. Dr. Scheatzle allegedly claimed that he found that palpation revealed tenderness across lower lumbar paraspinal muscles with muscles guarding in low thoracic area. Mr. Kirkman said that cannot be correct because Dr. Scheatzle allegedly never palpated his back. That is the first element of fraud.

The doctor's second claim was that Mr. Kirkman's skin was intact. Dr. Nichols in an interview with Mr. Kirkman asked if Dr. Scheatzle had ever touched his skin, to which he responded, "No. No, he never touched my back." That is the second element of fraud. Mr. Kirkman said he lifted his shirt himself so the doctor could see his scars, but the doctor never touched his back at all.

The next claim on the IME report, Dr. Scheatzle stated that Mr. Kirkman had no rashes or erythema.[89] According to Mr. Kirkman, the doctor never had him take his shirt off, so how was it possible for him to see if there were any rashes? This is the third element of alleged fraud.

Scheatzle did test Mr. Kirkman's Ranges of Motion, which is to his credit. However, the doctor went on to claim that in a neurological exam that Mr. Kirkman's cranial nerves two through ten were grossly intact. The problem was that the doctor purportedly never waved anything in front of Mr. Kirkman's eyes to determine if that was correct. This is the fourth element of fraud.

---

[89] Redness of the skin brought about by an injury or infection that causes the congestion of the capillaries located in the lower levels of the skin.

In the next claim, the doctor said light touch sensation was intact in the lower extremities, but he never had Mr. Kirkman roll up his pant leg to determine that. The doctor allegedly never used a pinwheel to test sensation in his legs and in fact, he never touched Mr. Kirkman's legs. Other than checking his reflexes he never touched his legs. So that is the fifth element of fraud.

On his leg raise test, Mr. Kirkman had pain going from his lower back down below his knee into his calves when he raised his legs between 30 and forty degrees, meaning he had positive straight leg results or radiculopathy,[90] but the doctor reported he did not. This is the sixth element of fraud.

To test hip flexion, the doctor only moved Mr. Kirkman's legs side to side, but did not have him bend his knees up to his chest, but Scheatzle reported that there was full hip flexion with knees bent, which is the seventh element of fraud.

In one last exam, Dr. Scheatzle claimed that there were no Leg-Leg discrepancies even though he never measured Mr. Kirkman's legs to compare them, resulting in the eighth element of fraud.

The length of the exam was noticed by Mr. Kirkman. Scheatzle entered the examining room at exactly 8:42 AM and the Kirkmans noticed the time when they were in the parking lot at 8:48 AM. For his time spent in the exam and for his report, Scheatzle was paid by the Industrial Commission approximately $350 to $450 dollars for an allegedly fraudulent report to determine functionality that stated that Mr. Kirkman was able to return to light duty work even though he was filing for permanent total disability.

The next battle was fought with Dr. John Stancil, a Cincinnati chiropractor who does file reviews for Corvel, an MCO. In his file review, Dr. Stancil said in his report that Mr. Kirkman had no flare-ups following his injury, but that was not true. Mr. Kirkman said "I have flare-ups constantly I have pain on a daily basis. It hurts like crazy." Stancil based his opinion by reading a handpicked file and did not examine Mr. Kirkman. He did not take into account the condition of Mr. Kirkman, with which Dr. Nichols takes exception.

When Mr. Kirkman first met Dr. Nichols, he barely could walk into his office. He dragged his left foot behind him. With Dr. Nichols' treatment though, Mr. Kirkman felt better and was able to walk with much less difficulty. Treatments were not always approved and the bias towards chiropractic care within the bureau was more than apparent.

Another major problem that exists within the bureau that greatly benefits everyone, but the injured worker is the practice of grouping diagnoses in order to get a denial for treatment. It is a win-win for the BWC.

Dr. Nichols described grouping diagnoses and how that works to the BWC's advantage. Using Alan Kirkman's case as an example, he said,

---

[90] Radiculopathy is a problem that arises with the nerves in the spine, which can emit pain.

"Grouping the diagnosis is when let's say the IW's claim is allowed for degenerative disc disease and the CSS sends the file to someone and he does a file review and says the POR is treating Spondylosis,[91] which is a non-allowed condition. That is grouping the diagnosis because Spondylosis is in the same ICD-9[92] category as Degenerative Disc Disease. Therefore, the treatment as in Al Kirkman's case should have been approved and not denied because the Reviewer was saying I was treating Spondylosis, which is in the same grouping category as Degenerative Disc Disease. But...the BWC ADR department, which supposedly reads the medical reports submitted by Reviewers or IMEs, should have known that the reviewer was grouping the diagnosis. They never thought about what that meant until I called them on it and talked to Steve Taylor. Think about the tens of thousands of IWs who had to go to unnecessary Hearings because these crooks were grouping the diagnosis. Al had to wait 4 months because of it and it happened twice. So he waited 8 months for Hearings." Considering the amount of damage that resulted from his accident and the kind of pain Mr. Kirkman had to live with, the actions of Corvel, the MCO in the case, and the bureau are inexcusable.

Dr. Nichols was hoping that Alan Kirkman's case would be treated differently, but it was not.

In discussing Mr. Kirkman's case, he said, "In short, the trauma surgeon told him that when the part exploded from the press it was in, it was equivalent to getting shot point blank with a high powered rifle! Baer and Soloman and the other reviewers claimed his injuries were healed according to their guides (Mercy and ODG, Official Disability Guidelines). They and the Bureau and IC Hearing Officers all violated the Tenth Appellate Court decision Reno Cameruca vs. Industrial Commission regarding medically necessary treatment, which says that treatment is medically necessary so long as it helps the individual function at a certain level no matter how lasting the benefits are and trigger point injections are but one example of this. The fragment was a wide as 5 nine millimeter shells."

Although the Tenth Appellate Court's decision was violated repeatedly by the IC and BWC, nothing was done except to throw Mr. Kirkman's case into more hearings and more delays, when he could have been treated. Instead, his condition deteriorated. Had it not been for Dr. Nichols helping him, he might have been in worse shape.

One of the more outrageous parts of Mr. Kirkman's case was a visit by John Ohler from Colfor to Dr. Nichols' office. Ohler was in the Safety Department at Colfor and somehow found out that Mr. Kirkman had an appointment with Dr. Nichols. So he waited to ambush him in Nichols' waiting

---

[91] Spondylosis is the painful condition of the spine resulting from the degeneration of the intervertebral discs. Oxford Dictionary

[92] International Statistical Classification of Diseases and Related Health Problems

room. Ohler told Dr. Nichols he thought Mr. Kirkman was faking. How does anyone fake getting hit from a two inch piece of shrapnel that lodged near his spine just two inches from his aorta? Nevertheless, that was the claim and showed Colfor's desperate measures for what they really were. They did not want to take responsibility for the accident and their goal was to deny Mr. Kirkman what was rightfully his.

With closer inspection of what Mercy Guidelines are, it is possible to see how the system is stacked against the injured worker and how doctors benefit monetarily.

Dr. Nichols knows how the game is played. He said, "The Mercy Guides were developed by a group of politically connected Chiropractors who were largely associated with various Managed Care corporations. They were developed as a 'consensus' of what worked best in Chiropractic office for the treatment of simple 'uncomplicated' soft tissue injuries. Uncomplicated soft tissue injuries heal in a certain time frame according to this so called group of experts.

"Their recommendations were based on their individual clinical experience that came together to form the consensus...hence the word 'consensus' that is included in the title of the Mercy Guidelines. Informal backdoor promises were made with Managed Care from most of the Chiropractors that were involved in this debacle. They were promised many perks from Managed Care such as routing tons of patients/injured workers to this consensus of doctors for Independent Medical Examinations, Peer Reviews and much more.... But the former were and still are considered the 'Steak and Potatoes' of working with Managed Care. Think about it...a Peer Review can be done in 10 to 15 minutes or less times 5 or 6 reviews per hour at a rate of $350 to $450 per review and your making $2250 an hour times 6 hours/day and your making $13,500/day times 4 days/week and your making $54,000/month times 12 months and your making $648,000/year and malpractice drops to nearly nothing.

"Now most people in the work comp system in Ohio and elsewhere who do Peer Reviews will argue that there is a cap on what they can bill and what can be paid out to providers who do reviews for their State comp system. And although that may be true for many, I would argue that these Reviewers and Examiners don't get the 'Steak and Potatoes' from the State but rather from the Managed Care corporations that can 'dole' out what they wish in order to get the opinion they want.

"Think about it: Managed Care corporations have doctors showing up for work, they're on the payroll doing Peer Reviews, but yet they are Independent Peer Reviewers? There is a stark contrast in what their role should be and what they are really doing right in front of the eyes of law enforcement and ethics boards who license these people. Many of these 'Independent Peer

Reviewers and Independent Medical Examiners' who render opinions favorable to the defense, can simply name their price for that opinion.

"The Mercy Guides were designed for uncomplicated soft tissue injuries. The Official Disability Guidelines (ODG) came indirectly from Managed Care, but here is the sham of both the Mercy Guides and the ODG guides: The ODG claim that all soft tissue injuries heal with only 18 Chiropractic visits, but the Mercy Guides extend that out to about three months. The sham is that all soft tissues heal the same. Soft tissues include anything that is NOT bone. This would include tendons, ligaments, muscles, nerve and etc.... Bones break and soft tissues tear.

"Here's the problem: When a patient has a soft tissue injury, such as a strain/sprain diagnosis, the tissue heals in three phases. First there is the Inflammatory Phase. This occurs during the first five days following a soft tissue injury. During this phase, the area of injury will accumulate more blood, swelling and inflammation, which explains why many motor vehicle accident patients don't really notice symptoms immediately following the accident. So it is not uncommon for the patient to experience a crescendo of pain following the 1st couple of days after a soft tissue injury.

"Second, there is the Phase of Regeneration; this can last up to six to eight weeks. So now we are at two months following the date of injury. During this phase the body begins to throw down protein glues or if you will 'scar tissue' to help mend the edges of the torn soft tissue. The patient may experience more stiffness, soreness and pain. But then the body moves into the final phase of healing called the Phase of Remodeling.

"During the Phase of Remodeling, the scar tissue begins to remodel itself, but this can only be accomplished with movement of the damaged area. The more movement applied, the better the alignment of the scar tissue along the directions of stress and strain. In other words, the scar tissue tries to parallel the normal tissue and the more movement applied to the damaged area, the better its chance of resembling normal tissue. This process can take up to a year to see itself thru.

"So it's easy to understand why many people have been diagnosed with strain/sprain soft tissue injuries and are still experiencing pain six months to a year later. Now it doesn't take a rocket scientist to figure out that these guidelines are obsolete. But here's the final nail in the coffin. The Mercy Guides do NOT apply to any soft tissue injuries that are 'complicated'. Complicated is typically defined as any soft tissue injury for which the Normal Timeframe of Healing is stalled or delayed. This would include such factors as work environment, home environment, pre-injury psychosocial and post-injury psychosocial experiences as well as socioeconomic experiences as well as a boat load of other factors that may delay the Normal Timeframe of Healing as outlined above.

"Every State work comp system has hundreds of thousands of soft tissue injuries wherein the claims are still open because injured workers still experience pain from their soft tissue injuries and do not want to settle those claims. Managed Care in the private sectors experience the same problems with soft tissue injuries...patients being diagnosed with strain/sprains or disc problems every time they go to the doctor for back pain or neck or shoulder pain on recurring visits. Soft tissue injuries comprise the most injuries in both the State work comp systems as well as in the private sector Managed Care in any state you travel.

"The paradigm of care (the use of these guidelines and others) has reached a bottleneck wherein the American public demands a better Standard of Care. Although the current paradigm is pushing its way through the bottleneck, it will eventually tire and begin to struggle as the American public demands a better Standard of Care. This is what we are now witnessing with the National Healthcare Debate. It is unfortunate that greed has led to our current situation. The current paradigm of care coupled with greed has costs millions of lives.

"Doctors should not be paid to do Independent Peer Reviews or Independent Medical Examinations for any managed care organization or work comp system. They should be required to be on a rotational schedule in order to maintain their status as a provider for such entities."

Mr. Kirkman's case and millions like his are a foretaste of health care in this country where guidelines like those above that hold true for not only chiropractors but also medical doctors. Certainly there are good and caring physicians like Dr. Nichols who care about their patients, but the problem lies in those doctors who sell out to the insurance companies. Under the new face of health care, we cannot expect more quality care. As it is now, quality care is becoming extinct and greed has taken first place for doctors and insurance providers. The sick or injured only have value as long as their illness or injury brings in the premiums and insurance monies and when those dry up or they have been on the books too long, they become liabilities. Without an extreme overhaul in health care, unlikely with the new legislation, Americans need to beware of the dangerous web that awaits them in the new and unimproved health care. Our chances of coming out of the health care system unscathed dwindle every day and the likelihood of being trapped by a humongous web grows exponentially. Currently, patients can still assert themselves in the medical and insurance process allowing for a chance at victory, but it is rare.

Alan Kirkman did attain a victory of sorts when he and his wife decided to leave the state of Ohio and move to Florida. Getting away from the deception and the cesspool the BWC he has found a new life. Able to move more in the warmer climes, Mr. Kirkman is able to play golf and to tolerate the pain he lives with daily.

Mr. Kirkman is not alone. A major migration is taking place. In 2007, United Van Lines said that 57 percent of its business in Ohio was moving people out of the state.[93] Ohio has been hit hard economically and the working class has been hit the hardest with the shutdown of many GM subsidiary companies and its parts companies. Other manufacturers, banks and clothing companies are pulling out of Ohio as well.

It was estimated that 36,500 Ohioans have left the state since 2004 and with them the state was hit with a $4.4 billion dollar decrease.[94] Companies have joined the exodus en masse leaving the state in an economic chasm. With state mandated Workers' Compensation insurance, companies can no longer afford to do business in Ohio because the BWC and MCOs premiums have risen too quickly outdistancing a company's ability to keep up. Even if a company could keep up with the burgeoning premium rates, the hearings and appeals process brought about by a broken system can inflict mortal wounds on even the most solvent. Someone should be questioning the efficacy of the BWC and the system as it stands. In spite of the political and financial advantages the BWC has for those in power, the system and the state are killing not only injured workers, but also any chance of attracting new business or employees to Ohio. Consequently, the house of cards, which corrupt politicians have built is about to topple and with it, the entire state of Ohio. The prospect of college graduates staying in Ohio and reversing the trend is unlikely. The workers in Ohio have taken the greatest hit and since the state's citizens are its greatest resource, Ohio is losing any accumulated wealth.

Although the worldwide norm is to decimate the middle class, it is up to individual states to choose to go with the disturbing current or to defend its citizens and particularly the weakest from all harm. It should not engage in the abuse of its citizens and profit from corruption foisted upon them. The sheer madness of institutions like the BWC that are given a pass by government will eventually ruin any semblance of order and annihilate any economic growth. On a federal level, unless health care changes and the attitudes of the elite change, this concept will play out against hundreds of millions of citizens and with it can only bring about the nation's demise.

Therefore, trying to balance the budget has been no easy task for Governor Strickland, who this summer changed his mind about bringing gambling into the state in order to create a positive revenue stream, but perhaps the better solution would be to fix the BWC or raze it to the ground and start over.

Even under the best circumstances, when Ohio's economy was not headed south, working in Ohio had been a challenge especially if a worker got

---

[93] Columbus Dispatch.com January 5, 2008 More People Leaving Ohio, Moving Company Says
[94] Brain Drain in Ohio? By Brian Kelsey. Civilanalytics.com August 6, 2008

hurt on the job. Governor Strickland has not been receptive to the predicament of the injured worker choosing to remain with his head buried in the sand, while innumerable workers are mistreated and abused by a system that he thinks is running just fine. He can see the problems with the state's budget, but he turns away from the solution to the entire problem, the citizens of Ohio.

There are far more injured workers within the system that do not fare as well as Sarah Shick or Alan Kirkman. Either through death, disability or migration, the state of Ohio has shortened its future and the future of everyone who still lives there. Sooner or later there will be no more people for the politicians and the system to rob. The poor and the sick will have given up everything including their hope in the air filled promises and the Madison Avenue slogan of the Industrial Commission: Justice for the Workplace.

In investigating the cases of injured workers and their contact with the Industrial Commission, it could be said that Justice has been a total stranger to its hearings and to its hearings officers. Yet, the same can be said of the BWC and to large extent its MCOs.

In the future, integrity would be harder to find as health care takes a turn into the dark chambers of the Marquis de Sade.

CHAPTER TWELVE
DIRTY LITTLE SECRETS

Sometimes the players in this game are so sure of themselves, so bold that they boast about how they commit their crimes. Certain they are above the law, these people explain just how they bilk the system and encourage others to do the same thing.

In a remarkable tape recording, Dr. Nichols actually captured one insider's crowing and posturing, which sums up the criminal empire of the MCOs and the BWC. If there were any doubt that these companies are acting above and outside the law, it would be dispelled quickly.

It is important to note that MCOs handle all kinds of cases throughout the country working with insurance companies whose "clients" are not just injured workers, but sick and disabled people.

Below are excerpts of one aberrant insider's diatribe and how she plays the game. As reference, MCOs like CareWorks have a long and shady track record of not informing injured workers that they are indeed a Managed Care Organization and Third Party Administrator or TPA, and that they have their own Vocational Rehabilitation company, which serves only the employer's best interests. This insider said, "Ideally the MCO for, example CareWorks, should notify the Ohio injured worker that they are an MCO, they are not going to offer to be a Third (3rd) Party Administrator (TPA) and/or they are not going to be a Vocational Rehabilitation company all in one. But this isn't the case".

She continued to explain how the whole thing is run against the injured worker. "Managed Care Organizations (MCOs) choose what they are going to do. The conflict arises because those roles outlined conflict one another because we approve our own bills.

"The incentive for profiteering lies in that MCOs such as our organization, CareWorks and other such as Sheakley, approve services that make the most money for our companies, such as the strategy of no DISCLOSURE, for example in the instance that we, CareWorks and Sheakley, who own or have contractual agreements with our own Vocational Rehabilitation providers or others, usually involves skimming-of-the-top, non-disclosure is the sacred phrase within the realm of our Case Managers.

"The guise is to portray ourselves as an Ohio injured worker ally or advocate. Unfortunately, this seems NOT to be our true intent in most instances.

"Training can happen anywhere in the Hierarchy of a Managed Care Organization (MCO) such as we at CareWorks or Sheakley who unfortunately for the Ohio injured worker, we desire not to forego training in the Hierarchy because our bonuses are affected in what's called Acceleration.

"Of course LT Nichols and others here along with other MCOs that share the majority of market share of employers were well aware that during the implementation of Managed Care in the HPP, Managed Care was not expected to cut the costs by 30%, in fact most experts throughout the US knew this to hold true. However, our lobbyists were successful in pushing the agenda in the Taft Administration in what would seem to be an endless stream of cash flow back into the Republican strongholds. Unfortunately the Cleveland Plain Dealer has exposed the reality of what we have so hard tried to conceal in our efforts to push our agenda. The reality is that Managed Care has doubled the cost.

"Interestingly, most of the lobbyists that were there during the writing of the rules for the HPP were from insurance companies and hospitals.

"Unfortunately, the rules were written to benefit everybody in the system EXCEPT the injured worker.

"So with this Hierarchy what we wanted to do, because we still get bonuses on things that happen and things that happen in Voc Rehab…our bonuses are based on from the time we open the Voc Rehab file to the time it closes…the amount of time the bonus is paid is based upon the least amount of time a particular case stays open.

"So if an injured worker was recommended training…the injured worker is going to knick our bonus if that recommendation comes in, especially from a private, independent Vocational Rehab company. If it's from CareWorks and our own Voc Rehab company or someone such as Sheakley contracts with such as in the past, Parman and Associates …we'll simply transfer the file to another counselor within our organizations.

"The term "Transferable Skills" is a term that is usually debunked by we at CareWorks or others such as Sheakley. Unfortunately we are forced to litigate from a Case Management point with Private Voc Rehab companies on an everyday basis because our policy demands that we position the term

Transferable Skills in our favor as well as the employer's. Our policy states that once we see this in a Voc Rehab plan, we use these words to deny 'training' plans but as odd as it may sound…our Case Managers really are not familiar with 'Transferable Skills' because of the Hierarchy. The methodology we prefer is to cite unskilled jobs that Ohio's injured workers don't need skills to do as a reason to deny the legitimate independent private Vocational Rehab plan. This seems to benefit our organization in most instances.

"Ideally the Hierarchy should be clear in that if the previous employer is not going to bring the injured worker (IW) back or if the IW has the aptitude and is willing and able, then 'Transferable Skills' training should be afforded to anyone who has the aptitude and desire to do so, which is permitted up to two years. However, this DOES NOT generate revenue for us and others who have a working relationship with Voc Rehab companies. If a Voc Rehab company does this, they have gone off the grid and it's time to either get them back in sync or locate another Voc Rehab that aligns with our ideology.

"We will cite that an injured worker has communication skills and that they can get a telemarketing job for six dollars/hour. We have to stay in line with the time-line or we risk the incentive bonus and nobody wants that.

"It's not uncommon to deny the Independent Voc Rehab counselor's plan for 'Transferable Skills' training, because it can drive the claim into Hearings that can take up to six months to process. There's a benefit here for us."

Unfortunately, this ideology is carried out throughout health care in the United States and will only worsen under the new provisions. The illusion that the new health care bill will make inroads in health care is really unfounded. With mindsets described above, the temptation to sell out a patient in deference to bonuses is too great.

The insider continued to explain the benefits of profiteering: "Our policy at CareWorks, until recently, has traditionally been to refer cases that we manage into CareWorks Voc Rehab, its out sister company why wouldn't we? The advantage is twofold for us in that we can successfully take the experience rating off the employer and transfer the cost to the BWC Surplus Fund where the experience rating is lifted from the employer. In other words, we simply flip the experience from the employer to the BWC Surplus Fund. It's just that simple. So we get paid for managing the claim as well as putting the injured worker through a CareWorks Voc Rehab plan.

"The interesting thing is that attorneys don't get paid if the injured worker is in Voc Rehab. A lot of attorneys are not going to pay attention to Voc Rehab because they make NO money if the IW is in such a plan so our job is push as many clients into our plans.

"We at CareWorks refer over 90% of our Voc Rehab to our sister company VocWorks. The money is good but the downside is that over time there seems to be an overwhelming sense of guilt in knowing that we really aren't providing adequate services but more like a glorified job search having

IWs searching the Sunday classifieds just to get a job any job for that matter. We are up against time lines for bonus incentives. Get the file closed is priority one. I can earn over $100,000.00/year. It is not uncommon for a case manager to put in nearly ninety-six hours/week, without discretion, we're approving our own services."

Such racketeering has caught the eye of some attorneys who feel that the BWC, the MCOs and the file review doctors should have RICO charges brought against them. One pending case in Michigan involves United Parcel Service and Liberty Mutual insurance.

The case questions the methodology of Liberty and UPS in their usage of "Cut-off" doctors who override Physician of Record diagnoses and write favorable reports for UPS and Liberty whereby the companies use those bought and paid for statements to cut off benefits of injured workers.

In the case, it is alleged that Liberty, UPS and other defendants used the US Mail to notify individual plaintiffs in the case that they had an independent medical exam scheduled. The court documents state that "UPS and Liberty made hundreds of such misrepresentations to claimants in the years 2003 through 2008. These representations were mailed to plaintiffs. These representations were false, because the doctors, such as Paul Drouillard, were not independent, in that they earned tens of thousands of dollars, or hundreds of thousands of dollars, each year for many years in a row, from defendants and other employers and workers compensation insurers, doing examinations of injury claimants. Defendants knew these doctors were not independent but were in fact financially dependent upon them and employers and insurers similarly situated. Defendants knew these doctors would generally or almost always write a report stating a worker had no work related disability. These allegations are based on information and belief, and are likely to have evidentiary support after a reasonable opportunity for investigation and discovery."[95]

The suit further stated, "One or more of these persons or entities committed mail fraud, wire fraud and or conspiracy to defraud, in a repeated and continuing pattern extending over years, by fraudulently terminating or denying benefits, by writing fraudulent medical reports and giving fraudulent deposition testimony, by hiring a doctor such as Paul Drouillard whom defendants knew would frequently give false testimony and or write false medical reports, by failing to honestly and in good faith review a claim as required by Michigan statute before denying the claim, and or by fraudulently

---

[95] United States District Court in the Eastern District of Michigan SAMMY LEWIS, JOHN MILLER, SHAWNE HENRY,
CHRISTINE SINGLETON, DANIEL HONOWAY, DANIEL DIDONATO, ROBERTA CAREVIC, JANET CONFORTO, ANGELA JONES, and MICHAEL BELLEVILLE, v.
DR. PAUL DROUILLARD, a MI resident, and or UNITED PARCEL SERVICE and or LIBERTY MUTUAL INSURANCE COMPANY, foreign corporations

terminating benefits because a person refused to settle a claim for the amount offered by UPS and or Liberty Mutual. Defendants used the mails and wires in furtherance of this scheme, by mailing, emailing and or faxing Notices of Dispute and other communications."

Since Liberty and UPS are national companies, it is not a great leap to suggest that this practice is carried out in all fifty states and their methodology is also shared by other large businesses and insurance companies.

A list obtained recently reflects the growing movement to unite major corporations under one MCO. The list from Universal SmartComp shows high-powered companies from all over the United States that have joined the same team for their workers' compensation cases. With the unification of these powerful companies, it makes it far easier for them to use "Cut-off" doctors and game the system so that their injured employees do not get the benefits to which they are entitled. The companies listed employ much of the American workforce and their treatment of many of their injured workers is infamous.

Dr. Nichols thinks we are seeing something dangerous in health care with MCOs that have super companies for clients. He said, "Get ready for Universal Comp Care...it's an overthrow of the current system...state by state. You know employers have been railroaded as well and it looks as though they're tired of it. Unfortunately, they have the money and power to do what they want, but when an employee gets injured at work, soon they'll get shafted worse than they ever thought. Soon legislation through bought off Senators and other politicians by people like these corporate giants will allow them to do just about anything they wish to an IW. It's coming. It Universal. This is what comp will look like 'Globally'."

Dr. Nichols is not being cynical in his opinion. After studying the issues and observing the current trends, he feels it is blatantly clear where health care is going not only in the US, but also around the world.

Many of these powerhouse companies go out of their way to videotape their employees, have them followed and have the audacity to accuse them of filing fraudulent claims when in actuality the crimes that are perpetrated the majority of the time are those committed by the corporations against the injured workers, or sick and disabled employees.

Dr. Nichols had a patient who had a private investigator follow her and videotape her. That tape was accepted and viewed by the BWC, but when it came time to view IME doctors committing fraud, they have declined to even look at the tapes let alone use them as evidence in hearings.

This lawsuit and others like it should put Americans on notice and alert them to the crimes that are being committed now and will be committed with the new health care bill.

We might feel lucky that we are with Health Maintenance Organizations or HMOs, but the sad news is that HMOs provide even less care than other groups do because they spend the least amount of money on the patients. For instance, a low back injury is rarely treated with aggressive medical care. HMOs normally opt for bed rest. Their bonuses are derived by keeping costs down, whereas the MCOs get the real bonus money by shuttling their injured workers in and out of the system on a prescribed timeline. Costs have risen under MCOs in direct proportion to their huge bonuses.

States that think that MCOs save the state money when handling workers' compensation cases are deceived. In Ohio's case, the state fund collected $2.2 billion in premiums, but paid $870 million in medical costs and $1 billion in cash benefits during 2004. The MCOs handling the cases received about 8 percent of the premiums that year totaling about $174 million. The Cleveland Plain Dealer reported that it cost the state of Ohio $1.6 billion just for the pleasure of doing business with the MCOs. Since their inception during the 1990's, it is hard to find any justification for their existence, fiscally speaking, unless you are a politician running for office.

There is great unrest with doctors and insurance companies right now that are anxious about how much government intervention will cut into the practice of medicine and the controls that will be instituted, let alone the worry about net profits and the ability to stay in business. If not controlled or entirely eradicated, new methods of fraud will develop by some prostitute doctors and insurance providers to guarantee cash flow, and other interests which clearly would not be for the welfare of their patients or employees. Some conglomerates have already figured out how to beat the system.

Currently, under the status quo, American workers feel blessed that they are offered health, disability and pension plans, but they are completely unaware of the true intentions of many companies that have made practices such as in the alleged UPS actions and in others that will deny benefits or drag reimbursement out ad infinitum.

One doctor who spoke with Dr. Nichols about how these major corporations work knew firsthand about corporate shenanigans.

In a taped interview with Dr. Nichols, this doctor revealed that he had done IME exams for MCOs. The doctor was a former US Army doctor, who worked for General Motors and other well-known corporations and in the course of his career spanning nearly four decades, he did IME exams. Dr. Nichols asked him if companies falsified their reports against injured workers to which the doctor replied, "Absolutely they'll falsify reports."

The doctor had firsthand knowledge of how many high profile companies and MCOs operate. He has even been threatened by them to change his findings, which he would not do. Apparently, he was asked to alter his findings on a regular basis by MCOs.

Dr. Nichols asked him if he handled any workers' compensation cases and the doctor said, "I don't do workmen's' compensation because I believe it is a corrupt system. It couldn't be more corrupt."

In his career, the doctor said he was very "vociferous" in lodging complaints against the system. "I really spoke out," when it came to corruption. Currently, the doctor is involved with a lawsuit that he hopes will turn things around, but so far, his complaints have had no impact.

Dr. Nichols has had no luck in getting the proper authorities to take the criminal actions within these organizations seriously. If we look at the statement made by the CareWorks insider who said, "Our lobbyists were successful in pushing the agenda in the Taft Administration in what would seem to be an endless stream of cash flow back into the Republican strongholds," the same must be said of the democratic regime now in power because it is uninterested in pursuing and prosecuting the criminals.

It would make common sense for the medical and chiropractic boards to go after their prostitute doctors, but nothing has been done and so the prostitution continues. The BWC and the MCOs know the vital role these doctors play in their scheme and have put pressure on governing boards to allow the criminal doctors to continue.

In a recent phone call to the investigative unit at the Industrial Commission, Dr. Nichols spoke with Scott Lape who told him that to his knowledge not one IME doctor has been prosecuted for filing falsified medical reports. Dr. Nichols pointed out that some Hearing Officers have willfully used falsified reports in their decision making process even after they were informed that the doctors' reports were indeed falsified and still rendered their decisions on those corrupt findings. Those Hearings Officers refused to view any videos proving those assertions.

Consequently, with exhausted financial resources, injured workers are forced to go to other government agencies for welfare, food stamps and any other help they can get, which means the BWC saves its money and impels other government agencies to pick up the tab. The taxpayer takes an even greater hit and the ranks of those on public assistance swell.

Polarization between the classes will widen and as the new health care bill goes into effect, America will morph into a socialistic nation and eventually eliminate our choices not only in health care, but in all areas of life. This has been the plan for well over 100 years and those calling the plays have made huge inroads using health care reform. We can anticipate that vaccinations for whatever disease either naturally occurring or manmade will be mandated along with other forms of medical treatments, which were not designed to cure but rather to eliminate Americans. Dr. Nichols was right when he said this was just the beginning.

CHAPTER THIRTEEN
BANKRUPTCY

America has been a victim of corporate medicine since the Nixon Administration pushed the idea of MCOs, Preferred Provider Organizations or PPOs and HMOs. It all started when Edgar Kaiser approached John Ehrlichman, who was the assistant to President Nixon on Domestic Affairs. Ehrlichman said, "Edgar Kaiser is running Permanente for profit and the reason he can do it, I had Edgar Kaiser come in and talk to me about this and I went into it in some depth. All the incentives are toward less medical care because the less care they give them, the more money they make."[96]

Nixon thought it was a great idea, so much so that the following day he scheduled an announcement to the American public. He told Americans he was starting a new plan of medical care for the United States and that he wanted each and every American to receive the best care even though he knew we would not receive it.[97]

Since then HMOs and MCOs have taken root and consequently we have seen the worst medical care in this country. It has been progressively getting worse because of the corporate medicine strategy. Therefore, people are not healthier in this country. In many cases, the standard of care is appalling. People are dying, as we have discovered just within the BWC system. The only positive things that have arisen out of corporate health care have only been realized by the amoral people running it. The only thing Americans have gained from the lack of health care is an overabundance of prescriptions that in most cases do

---

[96] Nixon White House tapes for February 17, 1971.
[97] Richard M. Nixon White House tapes February 17, 1971 and February 18, 1971.

more harm than good. Americans live shorter lives than our Western counterparts. Americans are sicker than our counterparts and too many Americans die waiting to be treated, arguments used by opponents of socialized medicine, but it is the picture of the health care now and it will be the picture of it in the future.

The new health care reform is not going to change medical care for the better, it will only get worse and it will use the mechanisms that are already in place in the MCOs and HMOS, mechanisms that lead to unwarranted and excessive death tolls, higher costs and burgeoning addictions to overprescribed medications to guarantee our complacency.

Like the review doctors within the BWC system, the doctors in the HMOs have mandatory high denial rates and like the BWC they must have no consciences. One doctor could no longer handle the guilt of her job. Dr. Linda Peeno testified before Congress on May 30, 1996 during a review of Managed Health Care standards. Dr. Peeno said that the more denials she gave the higher her income would be, which she testified was well into six figures. She received healthy bonuses for keeping costs down for Humana, the managed health care conglomerate for whom she worked, although they now deny she was ever on the "payroll." Her copious denials were exactly what Humana demanded from her.

In time, those denials had a significant impact on her conscience. One file came up for her review involving a man who needed surgery that would cost Humana $500,000. Dr. Peeno denied the claim and the man died. No longer able to stomach being a Lord High Executioner, she blew the whistle on the system, but like the BWC and in spite of those hearings, HMOs continue to issue their death sentences for the sake of the bottom line.

Dr. Peeno stated that she had to "use my medical expertise for the organization for which I worked."

She further said, "I contend that 'managed care,' as we know it, is inherently unethical in its organization and operation. Furthermore, I maintain that we have an industry which can only exist through flagrant ethical violations against individuals and the public."

Drug companies also acquired more power and influence and the result has not been positive, as the MCO situation in Ohio clearly showed. In effect, these corporations took medicine out of the hands of doctors and took control of a system that has been effectively ruined by them. Costs have skyrocketed in the 35-40 years of their existence and as result, more people are not getting the medical care they need and those who do have health insurance are not able to keep up with the premiums. Deductibles grow every year and the average family has no way to pay the premiums and the higher deductibles, especially in today's economy.

Congressman Ron Paul of Texas, who is also a physician, said that when he first practiced medicine, which was before Medicare and Medicaid that patients had more access to care. Doctors worked out their fees with their patients because the focus of medicine was on the patient and his/her wellbeing. The competition between doctors kept prices contained because patients had more choice about what physician to see and hence it was a patient driven system. During that time, patients paid the least possible amount for health care.

Consumers were not given a short list of questionable practitioners by their MCOs, PPOs or HMOs and told that they were the only doctors that could be seen under their health plan. The whole industry was turned upside down and if you consider the players involved and their associations with elite groups, the changeover from private medicine to corporate medicine was no accident. Neither were the failures that resulted from the managed care push.

Things are changing in an even more dangerous direction under the new health care bill, which is designed to annihilate the private medical sector entirely. Although we hear protestations to the contrary, if we look at the bill, private insurers will be pushed out of the picture entirely forcing the whole country into a single payer system run by the government. At best, private insurers could become a store front giving the appearance of a competitive market, but they will be phased out.

The unrest and deep concern in the medical community is obvious. Understandable worry about the privacy of medical records of a government run system is at the top of the Major Concerns List.

President Obama has made conflicting statements regarding the possibility of a single payer government run insurance program. In 2007, before he was president, he said that the new system should be set up that allowed someone to go to state and federal insurance and ultimately do away with employer coverage "a decade out, 15 or 20 years out." That backed up his statements at an AFL-CIO conference in 2003 where he talked about "universal single payer health care coverage." He was consistent and adamant about his position.

During the recent health care debate, he denied that his goal was a single payer government run system and that the government was not going to push out the private sector in order to take over health insurance. Did he change his position along the way? No, he merely cloaked his intentions. The bill speaks for itself and one of the president's supporters, Barney Frank, of Massachusetts, summed up the president's intentions on July 27, 2009 that "If we get a good public option, it could lead to single payer. That's the best way to reach single payer."

Single payer government insurance is where we are headed and although it might seem like a good idea; let us see if that is really the case.

Many Americans feel that the government owes us health care and in a perfect world not run by dark agendas that might be true. We should have the best health care in the world, but the best for everyone in the country not just a select few. No one should decide about our care but our physicians. Yet, we will not see that kind of health care. We will get care similar to what the BWC gives out and with treatments having to be approved. What are our chances of quality care?

Below are some recent figures within the BWC system where the word denial means cost effectiveness, but could also mean death for the injured workers. These figures are for chiropractors who did IME exams.

Collected BWC/MCO Reviews

Robert Blank DC Reviews

Sprandel Reviews – 188 reviews

1.   181 denials

2.   7 approvals

Todd Conley DC Reviews

Sprandel Reviews – 120

1.   115 denials

2.   5 approvals

Collected DC Reviews – 176

1.   149 denials/negative

2.   19 approvals

Tom Yankush DC Reviews

Collected DC Yankush reviews – 1063

1.   789 denials/negative

2.   274 approvals

John Hurley DC Reviews

Sprandel DC Reviews - 57

1.   47 denials/negative

2.   10 approvals

Collected DC Reviews – 78

1.   41 denials/negative

2.   35 approvals

Charles Lindquist DC Reviews	John Beltz DC Reviews
Sprandel DC Reviews – 35	Collected DC reviews – 71
1. 34 denials/negative	1. 64 denials/negative
2. 01 approvals	2. 07 approvals
Collected DC Reviews – 184	
1. 173 denials/negative	
2. 12 approvals	

The BWC saves a great deal of money with file reviewers like the aforementioned, and so do the HMOs, but costs continue to rise in spite of very few people being treated. According to experts who have studied the health bills, that would not change because there is no set budget and no one is really sure how much all of this is really going to cost. We have been told $1.2 trillion, but that figure cannot be maintained under the new provisions. Actuarial risk assessments will be a thing of the past and the federal government will be allowed to operate under its unfettered fiat.

Under the new bill, we will see a disturbing disparity between the government and private insurers. Private insurers have to have a capital reserve fund set aside to handle medical claims, but the US government does not. That is a formula not only for failure, but also the opportunity for more corruption, which will guarantee that Americans will not be treated fairly.

Further, the government will not pay taxes on the premiums they receive, as their counterparts in the private sector pay now. This should not surprise Americans. The government will not have to account for its payroll and benefits for employees, something which private insurers must do. Perhaps the worst part of a single payer government run plan would be that the government would set the price for services. Doctors and hospitals would have no choice but to accept those fees, like they do now from Medicaid and Medicare that slice fees by 20 percent off the top. Patients would have no input and the market would be destroyed. Additionally, costs would be passed on to other patients not insured by the government.

It is also quite likely, according to actuaries who discussed their findings with Congressman Ryan from Wisconsin, that at least 33 percent of Americans would be pushed off private policies three years into the plan. Under the insurance exchanges that are proposed, no new policies will be written after a certain period. That means that only people who already have policies are allowed to add a spouse or family member, but anyone new coming into the system will be bumped into the government program.

Americans are losing their freedoms on a daily basis. With the new health care plan, Americans would no longer be allowed to make a choice concerning their care and the kind of treatment they receive. The government would take on an ever greater paternalistic role deciding for its children and with that decision, America and Americans will lose the remainder of the principles upon which this nation was founded. We will have succumbed to the European elite mindset that it is better to give up liberty in order to be secure, a mindset thrust upon us after 9/11. Nevertheless, security is not in the overall picture and the truth will become extinct.

It is essential to examine how the Senate bill was debated and passed. Congressman Ryan said, "The House passed its health care overhaul at 11:15 p.m. on a Saturday night in November. The Senate cut off debate on its version at 1:19 a.m. earlier today – clearing the path for passage on Christmas Eve. There is something deeply disturbing about Congress sweeping through their increasingly unpopular government takeover of health care – one-sixth of our economy – in the dark of night."

For each of us, it is critical to ask why much of the crucial elements of the plan were not debated in an open forum. Brian Lamb, chief executive of C-SPAN wanted to know the same thing, especially since his network covered a great deal of the public debates, but was shut out in the final stages. In a letter that he sent to President Obama and to Congress, he said, "President Obama, Senate and House leaders, many of your rank-and-file members, and the nation's editorial pages have all talked about the value of transparent discussions on reforming the nation's health care system.

"Now that the process moves to the critical stage of reconciliation between the Chambers…we respectfully request that you allow the public full access, through television, to legislation that will affect the lives of every single American."

It will be interesting to see if C-SPAN will gain access to the joint debate on the bill.

However, as Congressman Ryan said, much of the final moves were made on the Senate bill in the dead of night when no one was watching or behind closed doors with only a select contingency making sweeping decisions. In discussing the true costs and problems for Americans, Ryan said, "There are countless poison pills in the thousands of pages of legislative text. I was most troubled to learn that over the weekend Senator Ben Nelson, a pro-life Democrat from Nebraska, backed off his efforts to extend the current law protections against the federal funding of abortions. In exchange for his support of the bill, all of Nebraska's new Medicaid costs will be picked up by the federal government – forever. Wisconsinites not only face serious Medicaid shortfalls here at home, but we're now on the hook for untold billions more to bailout states like Nebraska."

Unprecedented "deals" like Nelson's were struck that taint the very legislative process that has given birth to the Senate health care bill. The poisoned pills Ryan refers to will do more harm to Americans in the long-run and once discovered congressman and senators will be drummed out of office at the ballot box. The claims by the president and Congress alike that try to say that there are no taxes for people with this bill are misleading. The bill is filled with taxes that everyone will have to pay, rich or poor. There are at least 17 provisions for more taxes that will impact everyone.

It is also questionable that the Senate bill was ever read in its entirety before voting took place. Still, the Democrats were assured, once Senator Nelson got his sizable piece of the pie that they had the votes necessary to pass it. When it came to understanding the bill, few if any Senators had any idea. Too enamored with passing the "idea" of national health care, few took exception to what that health care would actually mean to the average American. Senator Nelson was not the only person to sell out his or her principles and constituents. The backdoor politics that pushed this bill through took Americans out of the picture and that was done out of necessity to disguise the true nature and the extent of the legislation.

The sad part is while Americans have been shouting about leaving health care alone, Congress has not listened. As a result, we will pay for it in the long run and our children, if they survive in this country will see taxation that will guarantee a much lower standard of living.

In thirty years, we could easily see people in the 10 percent bracket forced into a 25 percent bracket. Small businesses would take the greatest hit and would possibly see the 88 percent bracket. It is doubtful that this country will survive, if these changes are put into effect. The changes in the taxation is mandatory though in order for the government to pay for all of this supposed health care, which at closer look is a prescription that would easily shorten our lives.

In arguing about the demise of the lower middle class in this country, there is evidence to be found in the way the new health care bill is rigged. A single parent with children will likely not be hired by employers if a similarly qualified married individual applies. There is a mandated $3,000 penalty for employers that hire anyone in the lower income tier. The Senate's version of the bill means that the lower income individual would need a government subsidy to pay the premiums for insurance and that means the employer would have to pay the $3,000 just for hiring that person. This mandate would apply to employers with over 50 employees and make it nearly impossible for the company to remain in business.

It can also backfire for the employer by hiring a married worker, if that person's spouse is laid off or fired, which means the employer might be taxed $3,000 should the fired spouse join the working spouse's policy.

In effect, it is destroying prospects of employment for a large segment of the American population. Since the health care bill stipulates that insurance will be mandatory, this is the first time that Americans will be forced by the US government to buy a specific product. The only other mandate comparable is the Selective Service registration, but that does not mandate the purchase of anything.

Due to the high prices of mandated taxes, employers would be tempted to drop insurance coverage all together leaving employees who do not qualify for subsidies in the lurch.[98]

Dr. Nichols said he would not be able to afford insurance for his employees. He said, "I see a huge constraint on employers. As a small business owner, I cannot continue paying for my employee's health insurance because it would literally put me out of business. For large corporations their profit margins will fall as Managed Care strives to compete with the government run plan. Those who choose to travel the road of continuing to provide health insurance coverage for their employees will sooner or later find that it's much cheaper to just pay the fine and point the employee to the government for health coverage and show them a copy of the premium hikes.

"Managed Care will not be able to compete and the consumer will have no option but to look to the government for coverage of their health expenses. Unfortunately, the burden will fall back to the taxpayers of which will ultimately lead to loss of jobs as large and small businesses decide to pack up and move."

Obviously, the third party system of medicine has not worked as the MCOs in Ohio have shown and that means a major renovation of health care is necessary in this country. Still, the intention of the government is much like that of the BWC. It will dictate medical decisions, the patient and doctor will no longer be able to make informed decisions about a person's care. This unprecedented move provides an ominous warning as we have witnessed within the BWC system. Pencil pushers and accountants make life and death decisions, decisions for which they are categorically unqualified to make. Just as the BWC has not been stopped from withholding necessary surgery and treatment, the government will not be stopped either. As a result, millions could die because of this theft of American freedoms and it will be done without our consent.

The health care bills are so long that very few people have read them and that is what the government is counting on. The bill is filled with countless items that supplant the Constitution and many legal experts are crying foul.

---

[98] Section 1513(a) Senate bill on Health care

There are groups all over the country that want the debate to begin about the constitutionality of this bill. State Attorneys General are most eager to argue that there is no constitutional foundation for such sweeping changes that would eradicate Americans' rights and freedoms. Fourteen state legislatures are in the process of ratifying constitutional amendments regarding the bill. They have been organized and connected through the efforts of the American Legislative Exchange. Their goal is to ratify the constitutional amendments pertaining to the health care bill and would repeal it if possible. Senator Orrin Hatch and a member of the Family Research Council with a member of the American Civil Union jointly submitted an op-ed piece to the Wall Street Journal detailing why the health care bills are unconstitutional.[99]

The legal ramifications are just starting for health care reform that could tie things up indefinitely. There is an interesting side note about the Attorneys General who are behind getting the health care bills repealed. A good portion of the AGs have received healthy campaign contributions from the likes of Blue Cross/Blue Shield, major medical clinics, pharmaceutical companies and other health industry corporations.[100] Could their benefactors have something to do with their sudden interest in the US Constitution? No doubt. Regardless, they do have a legal point and without a major rebellion in this country, without the constitutional issues being addressed, our nation will no longer resemble a free society. Otherwise, government will continue to take control over additional areas of commerce until it has it all. Once that happens, Americans will lose the rest of the control we have for our own destinies.

In the United Kingdom, those that have watched the birth of the national health care system feel that the most important benefit is that a healthy society is one that cannot be taken over by tyrants. Healthy people speak out, protest and have no tolerance for a government that would try to steal its freedoms. Here in the US, that is another story. Apparently we are not well enough to speak out enough. We have acquiesced while the government has systematically taken our freedoms in the name of security and in doing so they have robbed us of our health. The BWC pushes people into pain management because it knows that a medicated worker is less likely to fight the unjust decisions being made and when the health care bill becomes law, we should expect to see a huge increase of people taking prescription medications.

The current proposed health care reform would unduly burden the entire country and by raising taxes during a deep recession, would not lead to economic recovery but rather complete economic failure. The federal government has no way to sustain the kind of spending it is engaged in currently

---

[99] "Why the Health-Care Bills Are Unconstitutional"
[100] Wonk Room January 5, 2010 Report: Attorneys General Challenging Constitutionality of Health Reform Awash in Cash from Health Industry by Igor Volsky

and certainly would not be able to sustain it once this $1.2 trillion reform takes hold without breaking the financial backs of the majority of Americans.

States will have a devastating hit if Medicaid is expanded because the already beleaguered treasuries will not be able to support it. Therefore, the states could end up being bankrupt as well. California, which is already in dire straits, might not ever recover.

While health insurance is vital, it is something that should be decided by individuals based on their needs and their ability to pay for medical bills. Removing that option makes it easier for the government to dictate other areas in our lives to the extent that we might be forced to buy only certain cars with the proper emission standards and no cars over ten years old would be allowed on the roads. This is another attempt to take total control of our lives.

The BWC and its affiliated MCOs have done their job in corporate medicine and provided healthy incentives to politicians to keep them operating at their status quo. We should expect the federal run single payer system to do the same thing only with a great deal more money.

In fact, the corporate medicine structure was a vehicle that was incorporated to take us down the road to a government run system and essentially had planned obsolescence. Corporate medicine has been a huge failure, but that was intentional. The whole purpose behind putting Americans in the corner over health care was to be able to control the population and what better way than without health?

Systems like the BWC and the government's single payer system are not designed to help people, not really. That is a worn out premise. They are in place to acquire as much money as possible under the auspices of compassion and necessity, which veil their true intent.

Dr. Nichols sees a depressing future for America. He said, "As far as what government run health coverage will look like: Take my word for it or not, but there will definitely be a rationing of care as panel doctors will review your claim file or examine you and they will be on the side of the defendant, the government. It will be worse than what we experience in the current state of work comp systems, which is a debacle, comprised of corruption and backdoor deals with no accountability no matter which state you reside.

"It's a business and will be run as such, but very poorly indeed from what we have seen of most government run programs such as Medicaid, Medicare and so on and so forth. Behind the veil will be just as we see with self-insured corporations with Third Party Administrators (TPAs) that manage the care of injured workers...and that is for their accountants to look at the numbers and deny medically necessary care while people lay in wait and suffer from their injuries or disease/illnesses."

In our dismal future we will have mandated vaccinations for man-made plagues, not plagues designed by terrorists as we know them, but by those people who want to limit the population. There will be no opting out when it comes to health care, and those who try will be incarcerated. This is not some Hollywood scenario, but something that has been in place for decades. Other changes have taken place in our behavior that have allowed dangerous people to take control of our lives. In effect, we have handed over our responsibilities and our rights to the extent that many of us no longer feel the need to dissent and those that do pay a terrible price.

America is bankrupt financially, morally and emotionally and unless we force accountability, unless we act, we are headed straight into the most formidable terrorist attack on America in our history, bar none.

CHAPTER FOURTEEN
MORAL NECROSIS

Many of us suffer from a degenerative disease that hits some of us harder than others. It is debilitating and highly contagious and now so common that most people are unaware they have it. Unlike usual disorders, this illness moves along much more perniciously as it infects individuals. Primarily the infection is almost indistinguishable to the person. In a sense, its covert nature can be deadly not just to the person, but also to those around him/her and once discovered, must be aggressively treated.

The disease could be considered a social disease by most standards and perhaps even more prolific than sexually transmitted diseases. Although you would not find that psychiatrists would mention this particular disorder because many of them already suffer from it and therefore their recognition of the problem is hampered. In the very basic sense, this disease is moral necrosis, and in a very strange and beguiling way, it is often sought after by those in power or those who want to acquire power.

We have seen it rear its cannibalistic head on Wall Street, at Enron and along the Beltway. Even the new administration, like nearly every previous administration is generously peppered with it.

If we examine health care reform, we can do a condensed form of research to understand where we are headed in this country. We only have to look at President Obama's health czar to get a clear picture that there will be no change in Washington and the clandestine nature of the deliberation process for the bills proves that Americans are not to be in the loop when it comes to their own health care and their futures. In spite of all the rhetoric and media coverage that talks about major changes in the way health care is handled in this country, there will be no great inroads. Instead, it will be business as usual and that can only mean a much higher mortality rate among Americans. Even now, our infant mortality is appallingly high, something unheard of in a developed nation of our wealth and expertise.

One would think that on an issue as critical as health care reform that the president would appoint a czar with an impeccable record, at least if you wanted to fulfill a campaign promise of real change. Unfortunately, that is not the case with the health czarina, Nancy-Ann DeParle.

With her record, it is surprising to find out that she has not headed the BWC in Ohio. Under her watch at several corporations following her first departure from Washington, she and her companies have been the targets of federal investigations, whistleblower complaints, lawsuits and a host of regulatory problems. Considering we are dealing with health issues, it should also not be surprising that Ms. De Parle was involved with health care companies that had serious kickback issues, but perhaps that is what makes her so suitable to be the czarina.

Illegal billing problems were also present while she was at the helm, making one think about the management of a government run insurance program. Already, before the reforms are in place, the country is saddled with someone in a key position with a tainted past who has seemingly succumbed to moral necrosis. There is a trend to put morally and ethically challenged individuals in key positions in government and the private sector. It can ensure a guaranteed outcome and keep their respective agencies or companies in black ink.

After running Medicare under the Clinton administration, Ms. DeParle headed companies that have faced allegations about violating the laws that she would have enforced while steering Medicare. The most interesting and dangerous aspect concerning her position as health czarina is that the companies she ran while in the private sector have a huge interest in how health care reform plays out. Citing the fact that DeParle reaped millions of dollars while working for these health care giants, it would stand to reason that she is somehow indebted to them. Yes, it is business as usual in Washington and as a result, Americans will pay a terrible price.

In the overall scheme of things where a predetermined path has already been chosen, we know how the government plans on running health care in this country. It replicates how the BWC in Ohio is run and then some. It is the same playbook with the same plays that always work against the claimant under the auspices of the greater good and/or "sound" business practices. For some reason, the people in charge of these programs and the people who appoint them to their level of incompetence have willfully skirted the law, and have suffocated any essence of the natural law that everyone has at birth. Is it possible that moral necrosis is that attractive? Simply put, yes.

Although people like Dr. Nichols have a difficult time understanding how people can mistreat one another for the almighty buck. It just does not make sense to him nor should it to anyone else.

Yet, the pervasive nature of the moral necrosis spreading across this country clearly shows that Dr. Nichols is in the minority, even if we refuse to admit it at first blush. If there were more people like Dr. Nichols that had a strong sense of right and wrong and who were squeamish about hurting another human being, the BWC would not have gotten as far as it has nor would the prostitute doctors have gotten rich. If more people were like Dr. Nichols, the corruption would have been stopped long ago.

Undoubtedly there has been a change in this country and the acquisition of killer instincts seems to be a necessity for getting along in the world. We have armed ourselves to do battle, whatever the cost, to guarantee that the Me in Us always comes out on top, no matter what.

Wars have changed over the centuries and as we have gotten further and further away from fighting in hand-to-hand combat, it became a great deal easier to kill our opponents. Strategic bombers and drones made it much easier to wipe out whole cities without seeing the eyes of our victims and therefore we became so far removed from the reality of war that it no longer bothered us or at least not to the extent that hand-to-hand fight would.

As wars became fewer, business became the new battleground and we changed our killer instincts to suit the purpose. Since the BWC and other agencies like it make decisions without getting to really know the injured worker or patient, it is much easier to deny benefits, to deny any help whatsoever because the soldiers making those decisions can do it from a distance. People become statistics and it is much easier to view a patient or injured worker as a meal ticket, a fraud, but not as a real human being with the same needs and emotions as the rest of us. Therefore, it is easier for those soldiers to make life and death decisions, thumbs up or down, and go to sleep soundly at night even though their actions practically guarantee a deadly outcome.

Due to the electronic nature of business and certainly within the confines of the BWC, people are detached from reality. BWC employees can lord it over an injured worker, whether consciously or subconsciously creating the mindset of the bureau against "them." To say the bureau does not foster an adversarial position with injured workers would be to deny the extraordinary amounts of evidence to the contrary. Bureau employees make their decisions by going through computer screens of data and making decisions that impact the lives of real people without meeting those people in person. The impersonal approach easily gives rise to viewing injured workers as third class citizens who are expected to "man up" and get a job in spite of severe injuries, but not until they lose their dollar value for the bureau, of course. Somewhere along the way people have lost empathy for one another and that is why national health care will be so deadly. It will make the BWC look like a house of mercy.

Americans do not realize that we have been dumbed down systematically and our emotions have been corrupted not only by our own selfish interests, but through media campaigns that have told us how to feel and to act. We must not forget those psychiatrists that planned on our behavior being controlled for any circumstance.

Very few people today want to make the right decision when it comes to the other guy. With the pressure within the bureau for employees and the prostitute doctors to have extremely high denial rates, jobs are on the line. Dr. Nichols' taped phone conversations provide chilling proof that empathy, sympathy and compassion for injured workers can rarely be found within the BWC's or Industrial Commission's structures. Certainly there are those heroic individuals who try to do the right thing, but those employees fall into a very high attrition rate.

Government run health care will be no different. The reform is not meant to make it better for Americans, but worse, not only on the health care front lines, but also in the overall picture. The reform is a means to an end, one that will not be a happy one for most Americans.

In the next few years, many decisions will be taken out of our hands whether it regards health care or other areas of our lives. By the time we awaken from our slumber, it will be too late to put up a fight or to voice our opinions, which could prove hazardous to our health in more ways than we can imagine.

We must take responsibility for what is happening in this country today, from the criminality within the BWC systems, health care and business. In some way, we have been a part of the problem either by sins of omission or commission. We have allowed greed to become the focal point of our lives. We have allowed the cheapening of human life as long as it is not our own and we have promulgated a caste system, which on many levels exceeds the brutality of those found in India.

It could be said that healthy people feel exempt somehow when dealing with injured or sick people. If it does not happen to us, it does not concern us. Yet, it does concern each one of us and hopefully we will realize that soon before all of our lives are changed for the worse. In a short time, people will wonder how the government got so much power. Just like the BWC, it became untouchable. Like the BWC, the government has found the opportunity to rape, to pillage and to kill those less fortunate and because proved too lucrative, there would be no desire to stop.

By allowing the corruption to be so well entrenched, it became the norm, so much so it made Dr. Nichols stand out as an anomaly, an enemy of the overlords in the BWC system and the one who was at fault and should be eradicated. That is what the bureau would like us to believe, and the federal government will try to do the very same thing. Anyone crying foul will be considered a crackpot, and eventually an enemy that will have to be destroyed in order to keep the sordid details from reaching the majority of Americans.

Not that we would raise much fuss since we willfully allowed ourselves to become impotent.

Somewhere along the way we have stopped asking questions, and worse, we have stopped demanding answers and accountability from those in power. Those that do have the courage to raise their voices, like Dr. Nichols, find that their lives are threatened and their ability to provide for their families is removed.

Dr. Nichols said he does not fear retaliation and the evil within the BWC and the Ohio State government. He believes the words in Psalm 23 and fears no evil. Perhaps Dr. Nichols suffers from an incongruity in society because he lives his faith. If he sees someone in need, he helps them – period. He fights for those who cannot, he treats those who cannot pay and has lived his principles, something that is now considered to be archaic, and stupid.

Society as a whole has become too sophisticated to care about spiritual things, about God and about helping one another. When looking at those less fortunate, we have forgotten that there but for the grace of God "go you or go I." Lying, cheating, stealing and killing have become the order of the day.

The best lessons learned are usually the toughest and it seems evident by the direction we are going in this country that we are overdue for some major corrections. By our apathy and our brutality, we have assured ourselves that we will indeed reap what we sow, a whirlwind of abuse, neglect and death.

A day is coming very soon when most of us will be treated like the injured workers in Ohio. It will be a day without rights, without recourse and without hope because we have failed to amputate the diseased limbs of our society.

The gangrenous stench of the BWC and the new health care system can only be masked just so long, but by the time we arrive at our final destination, it will be too late.

There have been remedies available to the BWC that would have leveled the playing field and reduced conflict of interest. However, the bureau never seemed interested in making things fair for the injured workers. All that is really needed is to move the injured workers through the system expeditiously, treat them and if necessary retrain them before they lose their desire or ability to work again. Naturally that would mean that the bureau and the MCOs would have to stop delaying treatment to ensure their profit margins and it would also mean that they could no longer drug the injured workers into emotional and physical hibernation where complacency is guaranteed and so are the big bonus bucks.

The system is gamed to allow review doctors to see the same injured workers over and over again even though that is against guidelines because the bureau would not realize the substantial profits without their prostitute doctors. The employees could become compassionate towards injured workers, but that would entail a major miracle and with spirituality and God being something nebulous to most people, that is unlikely to happen.

There are systems in place in other states that do allow injured workers to be fairly reviewed, treated quickly and put back to work as soon as possible, but again, the BWC is unlikely to adopt that practice because it would cut into its portfolio and returns. We all know how important those hundreds of millions of dollars are to the bureau and its MCO whores.

However, things do have a way of coming around to haunt people. The new health care reform might just take the BWC out of the game. State Workers' Compensation programs make up only about 2 percent of the overall medical expenditures in this country and that might not warrant Congressional review of the issue. Perhaps Workers' Compensation will be absorbed by the new reform, but it does not seem probable. Uncle Sam has to keep costs down.

Things will definitely change for the BWC when the national program is introduced. Although no one is quite sure what will happen, if states can even operate under the new guidelines or if employers will be able to pay their Workers' Compensation premiums and the penalties imposed by national health care without going out of business. Ohio politicians might be left stranded without their huge campaign contributions funneled through the BWC.

Employees at the bureau might finally know what it is like to be without a job, not knowing where their next meal is coming from and not able to pay their insurance premiums. They need not worry though. The government program is available and with it come the review panels and doctors that will decide if those former BWC employees deserve medical care, deserve to be treated like human beings or simply medicated to keep them quiet.

Yes, things do have a way of coming back to haunt us. Unfortunately, all of us will be faced with that lack of care and concern.

Will we be blessed to have a doctor like Dr. Nichols? We can only hope. Meanwhile, Dr. Nichols struggles with the critical issues that his patients face and struggles to find some way to bring attention to a major criminal problem in Ohio. He hopes and prays that the rest of the country will not turn away and in doing so fall prey to the BWC health care framework that will take over on a national level. Nichols lies awake worrying and trying to figure out what it will take to stop the prostitution and the crimes.

His health has been affected and he has had to make some changes in order to handle the incredible amount of stress that has been with him for sixteen years. Most people could look the other way and get on with their lives. Most people would give up after losing everything. Dr. Nichols is the kind of man who cannot look way, cannot give up when someone is hurting. The real question is can we look away? Can we afford to look away and to remain silent for much longer before this impacts all of us?

In New York City after 9/11, everyone pulled together. Differences were forgotten and people pitched in to help one another proving that we have not lost entirely our compassion and our ability to be charitable to one another.

Like anything else, unless we exercise that ability, unless we speak out and draw the line between good and evil, we could end up being the next in line to see a prostitute doctor whose only desire is to do the pimp's bidding. When you think how big a pimp Uncle Sam could be if we allow him to be, we best hope that society does not get any sicker than it is already. There is a cure for moral necrosis. It is simple. We only have to banish our lethargy and to use our God given intestinal fortitude and stand up and say "Enough!"

www.ingramcontent.com/pod-product-compliance
Lightning Source LLC
Chambersburg PA
CBHW060300290526
45789CB00001B/369